# BODIES OF
# TRUTH

Personal Narratives on Illness,
Disability, and Medicine

Edited by DINTY W. MOORE,
ERIN MURPHY, and
RENÉE K. NICHOLSON

Foreword by JACEK L. MOSTWIN

University of Nebraska Press | Lincoln and London

Acknowledgments for the use of
copyrighted material appear on
pages 175–77, which constitute an
extension of the copyright page.

♾

Library of Congress
Cataloging-in-Publication Data

Names: Moore, Dinty W., 1955–, editor. |
Murphy, Erin, 1968–, editor. |
Nicholson, Renee K., editor.
Title: Bodies of truth; personal narratives
on illness, disability, and medicine / edited
by Dinty W. Moore, Erin Murphy, Renee K.
Nicholson; foreword by Jacek L. Mostwin.
Description: Lincoln, Nebraska;
University of Nebraska Press, [2019]
Identifiers: LCCN 2018028388
ISBN 9781496203601 (paperback)
ISBN 9781496212658 (epub)
ISBN 9781496212665 (mobi)
ISBN 9781496212672 (pdf)
Subjects: | MESH: Clinical Medicine |
Disease—psychology | Narration |
Personal Narratives
Classification: LCC RC46 |
NLM WB 102 | DDC 616—dc23
LC record available at
https://lccn.loc.gov/2018028388

Designed and set in Minion Pro by L. Auten.

In memory of Brian Doyle and William Bradley

# Contents

# Foreword

JACEK L. MOSTWIN

"Considering how common illness is . . . it becomes strange indeed that [it] has not taken its place with love and battle and jealousy among the prime themes of literature."
—Virginia Woolf, *On Being Ill* (1930)

"The memory of an illness is very much like the memory of a nightmare."
—Joseph Conrad, preface to *Twixt Land and Sea* (1920)

You are holding in your hands a compendium of personal accounts of individuals caught up in the lived experience of illness, assembled by the editors for the public and the health care professions, designed to speak to the practitioner, the educator, and the general reader. It is part of a movement in medical education now called *narrative medicine*, seeking to restore a human voice to the experience of being a patient or a practitioner, and sometimes both.

In some ways it is a recent movement that can be traced to Reiser and Rosen's *Medicine as Human Experience (1984)*. A very significant contribution came a few years later from Anne Hunsaker Hawkins, whose seminal work on personal accounts of illness, *Reconstructing Illness: Studies in Pathography*, appeared in 1993 while she was working at Penn State. Hawkins sorted some 180 patient accounts found in book form according to illnesses, but, more importantly, she provided a much-needed critical analysis, examining the myths and social assumptions that patients employed to make sense of their conditions. Most importantly, however, she directed attention to the genre itself, distinguishing it from clinical case reports, seeking to restore "a voice to the patient," an objective shared by Arthur Kleinmann, Robert Coles, Arthur Frank, Rita Charon, Brian Hurwitz, Trisha Greenhalgh, and others in their advocacy for greater attention to patient narratives.

These narratives can be considered a subgenre of a broader literary domain called *life writing*, a term first used by Virginia Woolf, now bringing together categories that were formerly separated: biography, autobiography, and, more recently, memoir. Patients write for a variety of reasons. Some are already writers, and writing is what they do to communicate or to make sense of things. Some set out to create the book or memoir they wish they could have had available when they first became ill. Others write to help imagined fellow sufferers, or to provide a personal catharsis, fulfilling a primal need to tell one's tale.

Long before its more recent application to medical education, narrative served as an ancient literary form addressing ancient needs. We still hear the voice of Odysseus gathering listeners around the hearth as he pauses en route to his own kingdom. In ancient legends and the many memoirs and biographies that endure, meaning and value are transmitted by secret codes embedded in narrative, one form of cognitive structure that enables us to make sense of things. Who has not been mesmerized by such life stories at one time or another? Who has not felt the need to tell the tale? It is one of our earliest personal forms of expression in language. Perhaps when we were very little we might have come home from school, our faces full of joy or wet with tears, and been asked "What happened? Tell me," and then we'd start to speak into that face of genuine sympathy that we seek in our most personal moments.

Like Odysseus, doctors embark on long journeys and have many tales to tell. Our patients affect us; sometimes they haunt us. We remember them. We relive the experiences we have had with them because something important happened during an encounter, something that mattered to us. At the end of *Reconstructing Illness*, Hawkins added the following:

> Another voice we need to hear is that of the physician. This may seem a paradoxical statement at the end of a book that so insists on returning the patient to the medical enterprise and so often contrasts the patient's voice to that of medicine. But the "physician's voice" I am referring to . . . [is] the voice of the individual who is inevitably lost in that impersonal professional voice. We need to hear from them. . . .
>
> We need more writing that conveys the inner reality of what it is to be a physician in today's technological medical system. Only when we hear both the doctor's and the patient's voice will we have a medicine that is truly human.

What follow, then, are selected voices from these worlds that intersect in medical encounters. Some are very short, easily read in a classroom or on the run. Some are longer, demanding more time and attention. They are stories of what happened. They are not necessarily asking us to judge, to change the world, or even to react. They merely ask, as did Coleridge's Ancient Mariner, that we pause to hear the tale, setting aside for a moment the tasks at hand. How many of us have enough time anymore? Yet time and presence, the essential qualities of the listener or the reader, are what the narrator asks of us. It begins with listening, deep listening or patient reading, so that the tales can penetrate to the interior, allowing their secret codes to unravel within us and begin the unpredictable transformation so hoped for by the teller.

# Preface

"I knew that I would need to communicate during labor and delivery," Teresa Blankmeyer Burke writes in "Rendered Mute," an essay about the challenges she has faced as a deaf person and parent. "I *wanted* to be able to understand any instruction or encouragement given to me. I *wanted* to be an active participant. After all, this was my body giving birth!" And yet Burke was unable to find an obstetrician who was willing to go without a mask during labor so that she could lipread his/her words. "All I needed was to be able to see the doctor's lips. Was this too much to ask for?"

Burke's essay addresses a number of far-reaching issues, including disability, women's health, medical ethics, patient rights, parenting, and self-determination. Yet, like the other essays in this collection, it does so through the narrow focus of one writer's personal story.

Narratives have long been a vital part of medicine, and the stories of illness continue to circulate among patients, health professionals, caregivers, family members, writers, and others. As medicine continues to evolve scientifically, it also evolves humanistically through the study of narratives.

Discussions of such narratives are taking place not only in medical schools but in medical humanities groups in both urban and rural hospitals. All three co-editors of this anthology live and work in Appalachia, and we have interacted with health professionals in our home communities who are eager to find links between lived experience and literature. Many of them are family practitioners who see patients with every conceivable condition. While there are numerous memoirs that focus on a single medical experience, we found that there is a need for an anthology that includes a variety of voices and conditions from all facets of care. Because many health professionals have limited free time, we also found that there is a need for pieces that can be read in a single sitting. Thus, this collection came into being.

The essays in *Bodies of Truth* resonate beyond the healthcare fields. All of us have been—or will be—touched by illness or disability at some point in our lives. It may be our own condition or that of a loved one. Whether considering one author's dehumanizing tests to prove his neurological disability or another author's experience with infertility, readers will be able to relate to the challenges, frustrations, and pain—both physical and emotional—that these writers have experienced. The contributors are patients, nurses, doctors, parents, children, caregivers, and others touched by illness, disability, and medicine. Among the subjects addressed are cancer, cerebral palsy, multiple sclerosis, severe food allergies, death of a child, Down syndrome, autoimmune disorders, rheumatoid arthritis, depression, PTSD, and others.

In addition to relating to patients, readers will also be able to empathize with healthcare providers. From navigating the most basic interactions with patients—such as a handshake—to the challenges of staying current with pharmaceutical advances, contributors in medical fields take us behind the curtain of their professional worlds.

Because of the range of issues raised in each essay, we editors found it limiting to divide them into simple categories, such as "disability" or "ethics." In fact, since the very act of labeling is one of the challenges facing both patients and providers, we deliberately wanted to avoid compartmentalizing our contributors' experiences. We therefore have taken a more nuanced approach in determining the order of the essays, focusing on thematic connections and seeking a balance in length and style. It is our goal to have the essays speak to each other as much as they speak to readers.

"Medicine still contains an oral tradition, passed down in stories: the stories patients tell us, the ones we tell them and the ones we tell ourselves," writes contributor Madaline Harrison, professor and neurologist, in her essay "Days of the Giants." We hope to contribute to this tradition with *Bodies of Truth: Personal Narratives on Illness, Disability, and Medicine.*

Bodies of Truth

# Two Hearts

BRIAN DOYLE

Some months ago my wife delivered twin sons one minute apart. The older is Joseph and the younger is Liam. Joseph is dark and Liam is light. Joseph is healthy and Liam is not. Joseph has a whole heart and Liam has half. This means that Liam will have two major surgeries before he is three years old. The first surgery—during which a doctor will slice open my son's chest with a razor, saw his breastbone in half, and reconstruct the flawed plumbing of his heart—is imminent.

I have read many pamphlets about Liam's problem. I have watched many doctors' hands drawing red and blue lines on pieces of white paper. They are trying to show me why Liam's heart doesn't work properly. Blue lines are for blood that needs oxygen. Red lines are for blood that needs to be pumped out of the heart. I watch the markers in the doctors' hands. Here comes red, there goes blue. The heart is a railroad station where the trains are switched to different tracks. A normal heart switches trains flawlessly two billion times in a life; in an abnormal heart, like Liam's, the trains crash and the station crumbles to dust.

There are many nights just now when I tuck Liam and his wheezing train station under my beard in the blue hours of the night and think about his Maker. I would kill the god who sentenced him to such awful pain, I would stab Him in the heart like He stabbed my son, I would shove my fury in His face like a fist, but I know in my own broken heart that this same god made my magic boys, shaped their apple faces and coyote eyes, put joy in the eager suck of their mouths. So it is that my hands are not clenched in anger but clasped in confused and merry and bitter prayer.

I talk to God more than I admit. Why did you break my boy? I ask. I gave you that boy, He says, and his lean brown brother, and the elfin daughter you love so. But you wrote death on his heart, I say. I write death on all hearts, He says, just as I write life. This is where our conversation always ends, and I am left holding the extraordinary awful perfect prayer of my second son, who snores like a seal, who might die tomorrow, who did not die today.

# Spared

DEBORAH BURGHARDT

My mother falls in the bath, falls in the kitchen, falls on a sidewalk, so Dad tells a secret to me and my sister, Merry—nine and five—"Mummy is sick, you'll have to be *big* girls now," and I'm not sure why we need to get big so fast, not that I won't obey, it's just that Mummy doesn't look sick, because we can't see fatigue more severe than tired, an exhaustion that sleep doesn't cure, and we can't see that stealthy MS plaque, creeping along the spine, or breaking into the brain, robbing a person of sight or balance or breath, which in the end, Mum can't catch her breath, but I know there are people worse off than me, *me* who loses a mother at eighteen, after all, Mum is the one whose art will never be expressed, while I am left to dream on.

Merry rides a bike with both hands in the air, flies through the woods on monkey vines, and the time she breaks an arm, she doesn't cry, but I can see fear in her eyes—fear of the dark, fear of falling and getting sick like Mum, that is the scariest for my sister, who swears she will, but I refuse to listen, cheering her on as she swims to the furthest raft at the beach, cheering her on until I watch her drag one leg down the hospital corridor, whispering, "I want to die," as I try luring her into living with hopes of a medical miracle, promises of a life different from Mum's, and she says, "If one of us has to get sick, it should be me—the physically stronger one, the one who doesn't back down from a fight," and after she's gone, I wish I'd said, "You were the *biggest* girl," but I know there are people worse off than me, after all, Merry leaves Autumn, her seventeen-year-old daughter behind, while I am left to dream on.

And I do dream on, create a daughter, Amber—Amber with a mane of red curls, porcelain skin, a beauty full of dance and music and laughter, who starts to see spots before her eyes just before her wedding day, who finds she carries not only our woman lineage but the gene scientists seek, though she doesn't look sick, she sleeps and sleeps and sleeps, her memory fails, migraines pound in her head, and when she falls on the sidewalk I fall with her, clawing at that gene, trying to take it from her, wash it down my throat, and swallow it for the whole world—so it never falls into another body, so there is never anyone left worse off.

# A Measure of Acceptance

FLOYD SKLOOT

The psychiatrist's office was in a run-down industrial section at the northern edge of Oregon's capital, Salem. It shared space with a chiropractic health center, separated from it by a temporary divider that wobbled in the current created by opening the door. When I arrived, a man sitting with his gaze trained on the spot I suddenly filled began kneading his left knee, his suit pants hopelessly wrinkled in that one spot. Another man, standing beside the door and dressed in overalls, studied the empty wall and muttered as he slowly rose on his toes and sank back on his heels. Like me, neither seemed happy to be visiting Dr. Peter Avilov.

Dr. Avilov specialized in the psychodiagnostic examination of disability claimants for the Social Security Administration. He made a career of weeding out hypochondriacs, malingerers, fakers, people who were ill without organic causes. There may be many such scam artists working the disability angle, but there are also many legitimate claimants. Avilov worked as a kind of hired gun, paid by an agency whose financial interests were best served when he determined that claimants were not disabled. It was like having your house appraised by the father-in-law of your prospective buyer, like being stopped by a traffic cop several tickets shy of his monthly quota, like facing a part-time judge who works for the construction company you're suing. Avilov's incentives were not encouraging to me.

I understood why I was there. After a virus I contracted in

5

December of 1988 targeted my brain, I became totally disabled. When the Social Security Administration had decided to re-evaluate my medical condition eight years later, they exercised their right to send me to a doctor of their own choosing. This seemed fair enough. But after receiving records, test results, and reports of brain scans, and statements from my own internal medicine and infectious diseases physicians, all attesting to my ongoing disability, and after requiring twenty-five pages of handwritten questionnaires from me and my wife, they scheduled an appointment for me with Avilov. Not with an independent internal medicine or infectious diseases specialist, not with a neurologist, but with a shrink.

Now, twelve years after first getting sick, I've become adept at being brain-damaged. It's not that my symptoms have gone away: I still try to dice a stalk of celery with a carrot instead of a knife, still reverse p and b when I write, or draw a primitive hourglass when I mean to draw a star. I call our *bird feeder* a *bread winner* and place newly purchased packages of frozen corn in the dish-washer instead of the freezer. I put crumpled newspaper and dry pine into our wood stove, strike a match and attempt to light the metal door. Preparing to cross the main street in Carlton, Oregon, I looked both ways, saw a pickup truck a quarter-mile south, took one step off the curb, and landed flat on my face, cane pointing due east.

So I'm still much as I was in December of 1988, when I first got sick. I spent most of a year confined to bed. I couldn't write and had trouble reading anything more complicated than *People* magazine or the newspaper's sports page. The functioning of memory was shattered, bits of the past clumped like a partly assembled jigsaw puzzle, the present a flicker of discontinuous images. Without memory it was impossible for me to learn how to operate the new music system that was meant to help me pass the time, or figure out why I felt so confused, or take my medications without support.

But in time I learned to manage my encounters with the world in new ways. I shed what no longer fit the life: training shoes and road-racing flats, three-piece suits and ties, a car. I bought a cane. I seeded my home with pads and pens so that I could write reminders before forgetting what I'd thought. I festooned my room with color-coded post-it notes telling me what to do, whom to call, where to locate important items. I remarried, finding love when I imagined it no longer possible. Eventually I moved to the country, slowing my external life to match its internal pace, simplifying, stripping away layers of distraction and demands.

Expecting the unexpected now, I can, like an improvisational actor, incorporate it into my performance. For instance, my tendency to use words that are close to—but not exactly—the words I'm trying to say has led to some surprising discoveries in the composition of sentences. A freshness emerges when the mind is unshackled from its habitual ways. In the past I never would have described the effect of a viral attack on my brain as being "geezered" overnight if I hadn't first confused the words seizure and geezer. It is as though my word-finding capacity has developed an associative function to compensate for its failures of precision, so I end up with *shellac* instead of *plaque* when trying to describe the gunk on my teeth. Who knows, maybe James Joyce was brain-damaged when he wrote *Finnegan's Wake* and built a whole novel on puns and neologisms that were actually symptoms of disease.

It's possible to see such domination of the unexpected in a positive light. So getting lost in the familiar woods around our house and finding my way home again adds a twist of excitement to days that might seem circumscribed or routine because of my disability. When the natural food grocery where we shop rearranged its entire stock, I was one of the few customers who didn't mind, since I could never remember where things were anyway. I am less hurried and more deliberate than I was; being attentive, purposeful in movement, lends my life an intensity of awareness that was not always present before. My senses are heightened, their fine-tuning mechanism busted: spicy food, stargazer lilies in bloom, birdsong, heat, my wife's vivid palette when she paints, have all become more intense and stimulating. Because it threatens my balance, a sudden breeze is something to stop for, to let its strength and motion register. That may not guarantee success, as my pratfall in Carlton indicates, but it does allow me to appreciate detail and nuance.

One way of spinning this is to say that my daily experience is often spontaneous and exciting. Not fragmented and intimidating, but unpredictable, continuously new. I may lose track of things, or of myself in space, my line of thought, but instead of getting frustrated I try to see this as the perfect time to stop and figure out what I want or where I am. I accept my role in the harlequinade. It's not so much a matter of making lemonade out of life's lemons, but rather of learning to savor the shock, taste, texture, and aftereffects of a mouthful of unadulterated citrus.

Acceptance is a deceptive word. It suggests compliance, a consenting to my condition and to who I have become. This form of acceptance is often seen as weakness, submission. We say *I accept my punishment*. Or *I accept your decision*. But such assent, while passive in essence, does provide the stable, rocklike foundation for coping with a condition that will not go away. It is a powerful passivity, the Zen of Illness, that allows for endurance.

There is, however, more than endurance at stake. A year in bed, another year spent primarily in my recliner—these were times when endurance was the main issue. But over time I began to recognize the possibilities for transformation. I saw another kind of acceptance as being viable, the kind espoused by Robert Frost when he said "Take what is given, and make it over your own way." That is, after all, the root meaning of the verb "to accept," which comes from the Latin *accipere*, or "take to oneself." It implies an embrace. Not a giving up but a welcoming. People encourage the sick to resist, to fight back; we say that our resistance is down when we contract a virus. But it wasn't possible to resist the effects of brain damage. Fighting to speak rapidly and clearly, as I always had in the past, only leads to more garbling of meaning; willing myself to walk without a cane or climb a ladder only leads to more falls; demanding that I not forget something only makes me angrier when all I can remember is the effort not to forget. I began to realize that the most aggressive act I could perform on my own behalf was to stop struggling and discover what I could really do.

This, I believe, is what the Austrian psychotherapist Viktor E. Frankl refers to in his classic book, *The Doctor and the Soul*, as "spiritual elasticity." He says, speaking of his severely damaged patients, that "man must cultivate the flexibility to swing over to another value-group if that group and that alone offers the possibility of actualizing values." Man must, Frankl believes, "temper his efforts to the chances that are offered."

Such shifts of value, made possible by active acceptance of life as it is, can only be achieved alone. Doctors, therapists, rehabilitation professionals, family members, friends, lovers cannot reconcile a person to the changes wrought by illness or injury, though they can ease the way. Acceptance is a private act, achieved gradually and with little outward evidence. It also seems never to be complete; I still get furious with myself for forgetting what I'm trying to tell my daughter during a phone call, humiliated when I blithely walk away with another shopper's cart of groceries or fall in someone's path while examining the lower shelves at Powell's Bookstore.

But for all its private essence, acceptance cannot be expressed purely in private terms. My experience did not happen to me alone; family, colleagues and friends, acquaintances were all involved. I had a new relationship with my employer and its insurance company, with federal and state government, with people who read my work. There is a social dimension to the experience of illness and to its acceptance, a kind of reciprocity between self and world that goes beyond the enactment of laws governing handicapped access to buildings or rules prohibiting discrimination in the workplace. It is in this social dimension that, for all my private adjustment, I remain a grave cripple and, apparently, a figure of contempt.

At least the parties involved agreed that what was wrong with me was all in my head. However, mine was disability arising from organic damage to the brain caused by a viral attack, not from psychiatric illness. The distinction matters; my disability status would not continue if my condition were psychiatric. It was in the best interests of the Social Security Administration for Dr. Avilov to say my symptoms were caused by the mind, were psychosomatic rather than organic in nature. And what was in their interests was also in Avilov's.

On hi-tech scans, tiny holes in my brain make visually apparent what is clear enough to anyone who observes me in action over time: I no longer have "brains." A brain, yes, with many functions intact; but I'm not as smart or as quick or as steady as I was. Though I may not look sick and I don't shake or froth or talk to myself, after a few minutes it becomes clear that something fundamental is wrong. My losses of cognitive capability have been fully measured and recorded. They were used by the Social Security Administration and the insurance company to establish my total disability, by various physicians to establish treatment and therapy programs, by a pharmaceutical company to establish my eligibility for participation in the clinical field trial of a drug that didn't work. I have a handicapped parking placard on the dashboard of my car; I can get a free return-trip token from the New York City subway system by flashing my Medicaid card. In this sense I have a public profile as someone who is disabled. I have met the requirements.

Further, as someone with quantifiable diminishment in IQ levels, impaired abstract reasoning and learning facility, scattered recall capacities and aptitudes which decrease as fatigue or distraction increases, I am of scientific use. When it serves their purposes various institutions welcome me. Indeed they pursue me. I have been actively recruited for three experimental protocols run by Oregon Health Sciences University. One of these, a series of treatments using DMSO, made me smell so rancid that I turned heads just by walking into a room. But when it does not serve their purpose, these same institutions dismiss me. Or challenge me. No matter how well I may have adjusted to living with brain damage, the world I often deal with has not. When money or status are involved, I am positioned as a pariah.

So would Avilov find that my disability was continuing, or would he judge me as suffering from mental illness? Those who say that the distinction is bogus, or that the patient's fear of being labeled mentally ill is merely a cultural bias and ought not to matter, are missing the point. Money is at stake; in our culture, this means it matters very much. To all sides.

Avilov began by asking me to recount the history of my illness. He seemed as easily distracted as I was; while I stared at his checked flannel shirt, sweetly ragged mustache, and the pen he occasionally put in his mouth like a pipe, Avilov looked from my face to his closed door to his empty notepad and back to my face, nodding. When I had finished, he asked a series of diagnostic questions: did I know what day it was (hey, I'm here on the right day, aren't I?), could I name the presidents of the United States since Kennedy, could I count backwards from one hundred by sevens? During this series he interrupted me to provide a list of four unconnected words (such as *train argue barn vivid*) that I was instructed to remember for later recall. Then he asked me to explain what was meant by the expression "People who live in glass houses should not throw stones." I nodded, thought for a moment, knew that this sort of proverb relied on metaphor, which as a poet should be my great strength, and began to explain. Except that I couldn't. I must have talked for five minutes, in tortuous circles, spewing gobbledygook about stones breaking glass and people having things to hide, shaking my head, backtracking as I tried to elaborate. But it was beyond me, as all abstract thinking is beyond me, and I soon drifted into stunned silence. Crashing into your limitations this way hurts; I remembered as a long-distance runner hitting the fabled "wall" at about mile 22 of the Chicago Marathon, my body depleted of all energy resources, feeding on its own muscle and fat for every additional step, and I recognized this as being a similar sensation.

For the first time I saw something clear in Avilov's eyes. He saw me. He recognized this as real, the blathering of a brain-damaged man who still thinks he can think.

It was at this moment that he asked, "Why are you here?"

I nearly burst into tears, knowing that he meant I seemed to be suffering from organic rather than mental illness. Music to my ears. "I have the same question."

The rest of our interview left little impression. But when the time came for me to leave, I stood to shake his hand and realized that Avilov had forgotten to ask me if I remembered the four words I had by then forgotten. I did remember having to remember them, though. Would it be best to walk out of the room, or should I remind him that he forgot to have me repeat the words I could no longer remember? Or had I forgotten that he did ask me, lost as I was in the fog of other failures? Should I say *I can't remember if you asked me to repeat those words, but there's no need because I can't remember them*?

None of that mattered because Avilov, bless his heart, had found that my disability status remained as it was. Such recommendations arrive as mixed blessings; I would much rather not be as I am, but since I am, I must depend upon on receiving the legitimate support I paid for when healthy and am entitled to now.

There was little time to feel relieved because I soon faced an altogether different challenge, this time from the company that handled my disability insurance payments. I was ordered to undergo "a Two

Day Functional Capacity Evaluation" administered by a rehabilitation firm they hired in Portland. A later phone call informed me to prepare for six and a half hours of physical challenges the first day and three hours more the following day. I would be made to lift weights, carry heavy boxes, push and pull loaded crates, climb stairs, perform various feats of balance and dexterity, complete puzzles, answer a barrage of questions. But I would have an hour for lunch.

Wear loose clothes. Arrive early.

With the letter had come a warning: "You must provide your best effort so that the reported measurements of your functional ability are valid." Again, the message seemed clear: no shenanigans, you! We're wise to your kind.

I think the contempt that underlies these confrontations is apparent. The patient, or—in the lingo of insurance operations—the claimant, is approached not only as an adversary but as a deceiver. *You can climb more stairs than that! You can really stand on one leg, like a heron; stop falling over, freeloader! We know that game.* Paranoia rules; here an institution seems caught in its grip. With money at stake, the disabled are automatically supposed to be up to some kind of chicanery, and our displays of symptoms are viewed as untrustworthy. Never mind that I contributed to Social Security for my entire working life, with the mutual understanding that if I were disabled the fund would be there for me. Never mind that both my employer and I paid for disability insurance with the mutual understanding that if I were disabled, payments would be there for me. Our doctors are suspect, our caregivers are implicated, and *we've got our eyes on you!* The rehab center looked like a combination gym and children's playground. The staff was friendly, casual; several were administering physical therapy so that the huge room into which I was led smelled of sweat. An elderly man at a desk worked with a small stack of blocks. Above the blather of muzak I heard grunts and moans of pained effort: a woman lying on mats, being helped to bend damaged knees; a stiff-backed man laboring through his stretches; two women side by side on benches, deep in conversation as they curled small weights.

The man assigned to conduct my Functional Capacity Evaluation looked enough like me to be a cousin. Short, bearded, thick hair curling away from a lacy bald spot, Reggie shook my hand and tried to set me at ease. He was good at what he did, lowering the level of confrontation, expressing compassion, concerned about the effect on my health of such strenuous testing. I should let him know if I needed to stop.

Right then, before the action began, I had a moment of grave doubt. I could remain suspicious, paranoia begetting paranoia, or I could trust Reggie to be honest, to assess my capacities without prejudice. The presence of patients being helped all around me seemed a good sign. This firm didn't appear dependent upon referrals for evaluation from insurance companies. They had a lucrative operation independent of all that. And if I could not trust a man who reminded me of a healthier version of myself, it seemed like bad Karma. I loved games and physical challenges. But I knew who and what I was now; it would be fine if I simply let him know as well. Though much of my disability results from cognitive deficits, there are physical manifestations too, so letting Reggie know me in the context of a gym-like setting felt comfortable. Besides, he was sharp enough to recognize suspicion in my eyes anyway, and that would give him reason to doubt my efforts. We were both after the same thing: a valid representation of my abilities. Now was the time to put all I had learned about acceptance on the line. It would require a measure of acceptance on both sides.

What I was not prepared for was how badly I would perform in every test. I knew my limitations but had never measured them. Over a dozen years, the consequences of exceeding my physical capabilities had been made clear enough that I had learned to live within the limits. Here I was brought repeatedly to those limits and beyond; after an hour with Reggie I was ready to sleep for the entire next month. The experience was crushing. How could I only comfortably manage 25 pounds in the floor-to-waist lift repetitions? I used to press 150 pounds as part of my regular weekly training for competitive racing. How could I not stand on my left foot for more than two seconds? You shoulda seen me on a ball field! I could hold my arms up for no more than 75 seconds, could push a cart loaded with no more than 40 pounds of weights, could climb only 66 stairs. I could not fit shapes to their proper holes in a form-board in the time allotted, though I distinctly remember playing a game with my son that worked on the same principles and always beating the timer. Just before lunch Reggie asked me to squat and lift a box filled with paper. He stood behind me and was there as I fell back into his arms.

I may not have been clinically depressed, as Dr. Avilov had attested earlier, but this evaluation was almost enough to knock me into the deepest despair. Reggie said little to reveal his opinions. At the time I thought that meant that he was simply being professional, masking judgment, and though I sensed empathy I realized that could be a matter of projection on my part.

Later I believed that his silence came from knowing what he had still to make me do. After lunch and an interview about the Activities of Daily Living form I had filled out, Reggie led me to a field of blue mats spread across the room's center. For a moment I wondered if he planned to challenge me to a wrestling match. That thought had lovely symbolic overtones: wrestling with someone who suggested my former self; wrestling with an agent of THEM, a man certain to defeat me; or having my Genesis experience, like Jacob at Peniel, wrestling with Him. Which, at least for Jacob, resulted in a blessing and a nice payout.

But no. Reggie told me to crawl.

In order to obtain "a valid representation" of my abilities, it was necessary for the insurance company to see how far, and for how long, and with what result, I could crawl.

It was a test I had not imagined. It was a test which could, in all honesty, have only one purpose. My ability to crawl could not logically be used as a valid measure of my employability. And in light of all the other tasks I had been unable to perform, crawling was not necessary as a measure of my functional limits. It would test nothing, at least nothing specific to my case, not even the lower limits of my capacity. Carrying the malign odor of indifference, tyranny's tainted breath, the demand that I crawl was almost comical in its obviousness: the paternal powers turning someone like me, a disabled man living in dependence upon their finances, into an infant.

I considered refusing to comply. Though the implied threat (*you must provide your best effort . . .*) contained in their letter crossed my mind, and I wondered how Beverly and I would manage without my disability payments, it wasn't practicality that made me proceed. At least I don't think so. It was, instead, acceptance. I had spent the morning in a public confrontation with the fullness of my loss, as though on stage with Reggie, representing the insurance company, as my audience. Now I would confront the sheer heartlessness of The System, the powers which demanded that I crawl before they agreed temporarily to accept my disability. I would, perhaps the first time, join the company of those far more damaged than I am, who have endured far more indignity in their quest for acceptance. Whatever it is that Reggie and the insurance company believed they were measuring as I got down on my hands and knees and began a slow circuit of the mats in the center of that huge room, I believed I was measuring how far we still had to go for acceptance.

Reggie stood in the center of the mats, rotating in place as I crawled along one side, turned at the corner, crossed to the opposite side and began to return toward the point where I had started.

Before I reached it, Reggie told me to stop. He had seen enough. I was slow and unsteady at the turns, but I could crawl fine.

I never received a follow-up letter from the insurance company. I was never formally informed of their findings, though my disability payments have continued.

At the end of the second day of testing, Reggie told me how I'd done. In many of the tests, my results were in the lower 5–10% for men my age. My performance diminished alarmingly on the second day, and he hadn't ever tested anyone who did as poorly on the dexterity components. He believed that I had given my best efforts and would report accordingly. But he would not give me any formal results. I was to contact my physician, who would receive Reggie's report in due time.

When the battery of tests had first been scheduled, I'd made an appointment to see my doctor a few days after their completion. I knew the physical challenges would worsen my symptoms and wanted him to see what had resulted. I knew I would need his help. By the time I got there, he too had spoken to Reggie and knew about my performance. But my doctor never got an official report either.

This was familiar ground. Did I wish to request a report? I was continuing to receive my legitimate payments; did I really want to contact my insurance company and demand to see the findings of my Functional Capacity Evaluation? Risk waking the sleeping dragon? What would be the point? I anticipated no satisfaction in reading that I was in fact disabled, or in seeing how my experience translated into numbers or bureaucratic prose.

It seems that I was only of interest when there was an occasion to rule me ineligible for benefits. Found again to be disabled, I wasn't even due the courtesy of a reply. The checks came; what more did I need to show that my claims are accepted?

There was no need for a report. Through the experience I had discovered something more vital than the measures of my physical capacity. The measure of public acceptance that I hoped to find, that I imagined would balance my private acceptance, was not going to come from a public agency or public corporation. It didn't work that way, after all. The public was largely indifferent, as most people, healthy or not, understand. The only measure of acceptance would come from how I conducted myself in public moment by moment. With laws in place to permit handicapped access to public spaces, prevent discrimination, and encourage involvement in public life, there is general acceptance that the handicapped live among us and must be accommodated. But that doesn't mean they're not resented, feared, or mistrusted by the healthy. The Disability Racket!

I had encountered the true, hard heart of the matter. My life in the social dimension of illness is governed by forces that are severe and implacable. Though activism has helped protect the handicapped over the last four decades, there is little room for reciprocity between the handicapped person and his or her world. It is naive to expect otherwise.

I would like to think that the insurance company didn't send an official letter of findings because they were abashed at what they'd put me through. I would like to think that Dr. Avilov, who no longer practices in Salem, hasn't moved away because he found too many claimants disabled and lost his contract with the Social Security Administration. That my experience educated Reggie and his firm, and that his report educated the insurance company, so everyone now understands the experience of disability or of living with brain damage.

But I know better. My desire for reciprocity between self and world must find its form in writing about my experience. Slowly. This essay has taken me eleven months to complete in sittings of fifteen minutes or so. Built of fragments shaped after the pieces were examined, its errors of spelling and of word choice and logic ferreted out with the help of my wife or daughter or computer's spell-checker. It may look to a reader like the product of someone a lot less damaged than I claim to be. But it's not. It's the product of someone who has learned how to live with his limitations and work with them. And when it's published, if someone employed by my insurance company reads it, I will probably get a letter in the mail demanding that I report for another battery of tests. After all, this is not how a brain-damaged man is supposed to behave.

# One Little Mind, Our Lie, Dr. Lie

MATTHEW S. SMITH

Medicine, like life, is made up of moments. Their significance may not be apparent while you are living them but becomes clearer when recalled through the fog of memory. Here is a moment that haunts me, making me wish that I had done things differently—recording, storing, and enjoying its significance.

I was the neurology resident on call. I am not sure of the year. I remember it was late, I had worked close to twenty-four hours, and without warning one of "the aphasics" darted out of her room to accost me with a piece of paper. I was stunned by her sudden attack but too tired to attempt defense. She thrust the folded-up sheet of plain paper in my hand before disappearing into the darkness of her room, shutting the door behind her. I put the paper in my pocket to read later, not knowing what I might find.

Maybe it was youth or hubris, but I didn't think much of it at the time. I just wanted to go home and sleep. I had done my duty: admitting and keeping the patients alive for one more night while everyone else slumbered. I placed it in my pocket to later be deposited in the pile of detritus of partially read journal articles, bills, and "important" but yet unfiled papers.

It was one of those moments when you are searching for something else, and you stumble onto a memory that makes you forget the original errand. Maybe I was in a more introspective state, maybe I had been reading too much Oliver Sacks or V. S. Ramachandran. I unfolded the as-yet-unread letter from years before and found the following (transcription from the original letter):

### Dr Lie

They a bottle, is I hospital, I'm
The Vicodin, Lie Answer Numbers
They pain you pills, they eyes
They pains, wrote angry. I wrote
The pills as easy!
Dr Lie, as a lawyer as lie as
I needy not Dr? Lawyer?
Every??
Please are you doing she
Is mind—everyone little lie
You everyone!
One little mind
Our lie. Help!
Minds

I was struck by the poetry and rhythm of the letter. She was like the patients Sacks talked about in "The President's Speech" in *The Man Who Mistook His Wife for a Hat*, with the feeling-tone of Henry Head and certainly not like the dogs of Hughlings Jackson. She had lost her grammatical voice but had found a new one. A voice that was able to convey the confusion and frustration perhaps better than a typical essayist could, with her right brain now free to express her feeling in a poetic way.

I don't know what happened to this latent poet. She was lost to me the moment I left the ward, not even knowing who she was other than "left MCA stroke with expressive aphasia."

Her framed letter lives on in my office as a reminder of the mysteries of communication and as an admonition to cherish the moments of practice, because there are so many poignant moments and you never know which of them will change your life forever.

DR LiE,

LiE They A Bottle is I hospital, I'm
the Vicodin, LiE ANSWER NUMBERS

LiE they pain you pills, they EYES
they pains, wrote ~~ANREY~~ ANGRY. I WROTE
the EX pills as EaSy!

DR LiE, as a LAYWER as lie as
I NEEDY NOT DR-? LAYWER??
EVERY ??.

PLEASE ARE you DOING She
is MIND - everyone Little lie
you EVERYONE!

ONE LiTtLe MiND
OUR LiE . help!
MiNDS!

# Locked into Life

MARK BRAZAITIS

In a locked psychiatric facility you're obliged to keep living—unless, that is, you're extraordinarily desperate and creative about instruments of self-destruction: a half-pint milk carton, a Chutes and Ladders game board, a plastic spoon. Your safety and well-being are the staff's primary concern. If you're suffering from severe depression, like me, you may not consider this a benefit. If you believe your depression is incurable, you may even feel deprived of the one escape you had. Life is hard, and then you can't kill yourself.

In the autumn of 2003, at the age of thirty-seven, I find myself entering such a facility in New York City, four hundred miles from my home in Morgantown, West Virginia. My brother-in-law works as a psychologist in a different section of the same hospital and has arranged for me to be part of a group that receives free care in exchange for being available, though not obligated, to participate in experimental treatments and drug trials.

On my first day I attend Art Therapy. The eleven other patients and I click self-portraits with an old camera, then watch the pictures develop in a darkroom. The smell of the chemicals reminds me of the basement darkroom my father, a journalist and photographer, used three decades ago.

For most of my life I have feared and distrusted my father. As a young parent he had a temper and was often hard on me. When I was in elementary school, he once left the kitchen trashcan on my bed after I'd failed to haul it to the curb the previous night. When I was thirteen, he sold me his lawnmower for my budding lawn-care business but didn't refund any of the money I'd paid him when, two weeks later, it broke down. ("Looks like I got the better end of that deal," he said.) He'd been a college athlete, and when, as a high-school student, I veered away from baseball and basketball and toward books, he didn't hide his disappointment. As he's aged, however, he's become more easygoing and more interested in me. These changes make me hopeful about the future of our relationship. But now the kidney cancer he thought he beat a couple of years ago has metastasized, and he is dying.

I suspect my father's cancer is one reason for my recent slide into a profound and hope-killing darkness. Other possible reasons? The recent death of my maternal grandmother, who loved my poetry. A creeping sense that my two young daughters will inherit a world so damaged by global warming and terrorism as to be unlivable. My apprehension about my body's decline. Or perhaps I owe my depression only to the chemicals in my brain, which I'm told have become unbalanced, like a canoe in which one of the paddlers has suddenly stood up and stomped his feet.

When my self-portrait is fully developed, I see my father's chin and my mother's cheeks but nothing of myself. The art therapist asks us to use magic markers to color our black-and-white photos. I use a single marker: blue.

A recovering drug addict named Adam, who also lives in the facility, is mystified by my condition, especially when he discovers I've written and published two books. "You can't feel sad if you've written two books!" he announces. He prints pages from Amazon's website to attest to my accomplishments and tapes them to the wall of my bedroom: reminders of a life I'm convinced I'll never recapture. They only reinforce my depression.

Adam is my height (six feet) but ten years younger and thirty pounds heavier, with a fringe of black beard. He lusts after Erica, one of the nurses. He confides to me that when blond, buxom, soft-spoken Erica is behind the counter distributing medicines, he sometimes knocks his pills to the floor just to see her bend over to retrieve them. "You should try it," he says, grinning. I remind him I'm married. I don't tell him that if my sex drive were a car, it would be sitting on the side of an abandoned road, rusting.

He's glad he's a drug addict, Adam tells me, instead of a depressive. "Your misery," he says, "is worse than mine." I'm not sure it's so clear-cut. One night, while I'm struggling to sleep, I hear the heroin addict in the room next to mine vomiting and defecating with a violence I wouldn't have thought possible. His agony lasts for hours.

Before long Adam's affections shift from Erica to Emily, a twenty-year-old anorexic. Emily and her fellow anorexics participate with the rest of us in groups—Art Therapy, Self-Esteem, Readjustment to Society—but they must spend an hour after every meal confined to the dayroom, under a nurse's watchful eyes, lest they sneak off to the bathroom to throw up. As they show signs of recovery they are allowed small privileges, such as the right to visit the cafe on the third floor. The cafe is the site of Adam and Emily's dates. After a couple of weeks, however, Adam confesses to being bored. "It's so easy," he says. "She's so full of longing. They all are."

Despite their alarming thinness the anorexics are beautiful. Among themselves they seem to speak a secret language. I don't know whether it's the language of anorexia or simply of youth. None are older than twenty-one.

The Readjustment to Society group, whose name might have been invented by George Orwell's Ministry of Truth, is run by a short woman in her late sixties named Mrs. Edelstein. She wears glasses and looks as if she might once have taught second grade. One morning she asks each of us to recount something joyful in our lives. I can't complete the assignment. To conjure such a moment from my past is also to mark how far it is from how I'm feeling now. When it's my turn, I say, "I don't remember."

"You must remember something joyful," Mrs. Edelstein says. "What about the birth of one of your daughters?"

"After my second daughter was born," I say, "I sat in a chair at the foot of my wife's hospital bed and thought, Now I know who will bury me." As I tell it the anecdote seems morbid, and maybe unintentionally funny. But, in fact, the thought had been peaceful: My wife and I planned to have no more children. Our family was complete. Should death allow my children to outlive me, I knew who would be at my graveside.

Mrs. Edelstein looks at me with concern. "What about the birth of your first daughter?" she asks.

"I cried," I say. The session ends before I can specify that they were tears of joy.

Because it's a teaching facility, I see dozens of psychiatrists-in-training. I have the same conversation countless times:

"How are you feeling?"

"Depressed."

"Have you noticed any change in your mood?"

"No."

There's one exception. A month into my stay I am seen by a psychiatry resident who has a degree from Harvard, like me. Instead of asking how I feel, he asks what year I graduated, where I lived on campus, and whether we might know anyone in common. We trade names but find no mutual connections. It's the kind of awkward conversation I usually have with people at parties or conferences, and it highlights the gap between where, as a Harvard graduate, I think I ought to be and where I am. (Of course, more Harvard grads have ended up in the nuthouse than in the White House.)

During free hours, when I'm not pacing the hallways—the medication I've been given makes me unable to sit still for long—I occasionally participate in the residents' favorite card game: Crazy Eights. (Only much later will I laugh at the irony of our choice of leisure activity.)

The Recreation group is held in a basement gym run by a man named Pedro in his mid-twenties. I go there and play basketball by myself, pretending, as I did when I was eight years old, to be different players on a team that competes against NBA All-Stars. I revive my made-up dream team's players: Carl "Peanut" Carson, Alex "Shorty" Johnson, John "Too" Long. I imagine that the October light slipping through the gym's lone, large window is beaming from the ceiling at Madison Square Garden. These days I doubt I would win a game of twenty-one against my eight-year-old self, who would have the advantage not only of youth but of enthusiasm.

After several weeks of my lethargic, one-on-none games, Pedro hands me a pair of ten-pound dumbbells and sits me down on a bench in the weight room. He becomes my personal trainer, encouraging me and pushing me out of complacency and torpor. If I could I would lift the whole building for him. He's this inspiring. But, of course, I'm not inspired.

My wife calls me every day. One night she puts our older daughter, who is three and a half, on the phone. "I miss you, Daddy," she says. Irrationally, because depression induces irrationality, I detect both disappointment and reproach in her voice. I am sure I will be a bigger disappointment to my daughters than my father ever was to me. After the call I retreat to my bedroom, where I picture my depression as a boxing opponent. I swing wildly, furiously, desperately, until I've exhausted myself and collapse onto my bed. The next day I ask my wife about our daughter's comment. No doubt sensing my anxiety, she says, "Don't worry about it, sweetheart. She says 'I miss you' to everyone. Today it was the woman who bagged our groceries at Giant Eagle."

My wife brings our daughters to visit me in November, after I've been at the facility for several weeks. We gather in the family room, an eight-by-ten cell with brown carpet and a single window. When our younger daughter settles into my lap for me to read to her, I feel nothing but despair. I am convinced again that I am incurable, that my affliction will persist indefinitely, that I am a colossal failure. I am relieved when the hour ends and I am called into Group Therapy.

I eat the same meals every day: cereal for breakfast, a sandwich for lunch, chicken for dinner. I don't taste any of it, which is a commentary not on the food but rather on how dulled my sense of taste has become. Thanksgiving passes. Christmas arrives. From the facility's staff I receive a long-sleeved red shirt. They know me well; it fits perfectly.

My steadfast but frustrated wife says she can't understand why the treatments I've received over the past ten weeks have brought me no closer to my old self. "I think we need to consider ECT," she tells me over the phone one night. Electroconvulsive therapy or, as it's still sometimes called, "shock therapy."

Early in my depression I resisted even antidepressants, believing they would kill my creativity. As I wandered the corridors during my first week in the facility, a fellow patient—a middle-aged woman who had lost all her top teeth when she'd tried to kill herself by driving into a tree—pegged me as a candidate for ECT. To me, however, ECT seems extreme, dangerous, and destined to fail. (I've seen *One Flew Over the Cuckoo's Nest*, after all. Jack Nicholson's character doesn't exactly find happiness in the wake of his electroshock therapy.) But now anything short of a lobotomy seems reasonable if it will bring me relief.

My wife arranges a meeting with the facility's ECT doctors. My mother, my sister, and my brother-in-law are also there. I am too terrified and defeated to take in much of what's said. I understand there are risks to the procedure, like memory loss. And even after twelve treatments I might not feel any better. Predictably I believe this will be the outcome.

"I have no faith," I tell my wife.

"Trust mine," she says.

A week later, as I am lying on the ECT table, electrodes stuck to my head, the anesthesiologist notes that his daughter and my younger daughter share a first name. I can recognize his comment as an effort to make a connection, however slight, but in my current mental state I wonder how he learned my daughter's name and what else he and the rest of the ECT team know about me and what they might do with this information. He asks me to count backwards from ten. At three I'm out.

I wake up in a recovery room, my wife by my side, and inexplicably I start crying. One of the nurses blames the anesthetic. (Later I'll wonder if I wept because I'd recognized the remarkable: I was feeling better.) My wife escorts me to my room, where I sleep the deepest, most rejuvenating sleep I've had in a year.

I am told I should expect a setback or two—periods of darkness amid the welcome and unfamiliar light. But darkness never intrudes; what I feel most profoundly are relief and exhaustion. After each of my twelve ECT treatments I slip back to my room and sleep. After dinner, when there are no groups to attend or psychiatrists to see, I do the same. I am, I understand, catching up after months of mind-crushing insomnia. Sleep isn't just necessary; it's delicious and reviving.

Over the weeks of my ECT treatment I suffer occasionally from headaches. And my short-term memory is poor. I read an entire Louise Erdrich novel whose plot and characters I forget as soon as I close the book. Under different circumstances I might find this disturbing. But I am amazed I am able to read at all.

By mid-January, after my last ECT treatment, I've made an amazing recovery. I taste my meals. I see how fragile the young anorexics are, downing their bottles of Ensure and vowing to stop their clandestine nighttime exercising. But I also see how they're like other women their age in their reverence for certain movies and TV shows and pop songs. I lift more weights for Pedro and am, at last, able to thank him genuinely for his help.

I am well enough to receive an overnight pass—dusk to dawn

in New York City. My wife and I borrow a friend's apartment for the night, and there we make love cautiously, braced for failure—like Odysseus and Penelope once her suitors have been slain. The gods smile on us.

After three and a half months at the facility, I'm scheduled to be discharged. I spend my last night in the cafeteria with Rachel, who is sixteen and a cutter. She's devoted to books and ideas and reminds me of myself at her age. She points to the George Washington Bridge, which looms outside the cafeteria window. "Would you die if you jumped from it?" she asks.

"I think so," I say, then find myself wondering why anyone would want to die.

When I get home I will begin rebuilding a life I hope will be free from catastrophic depression. I'm aware there will be no guarantees, even with the antidepressant and the lithium I've been prescribed, even with the therapist and the psychiatrist my wife has arranged for me to see. Toward the end of "Sonny's Blues," the classic short story by James Baldwin, Sonny admits to his older brother that, although he appears to have kicked his heroin habit, "it can come again." So, too, could my depression. Sometimes even now, ten years later, I feel it, like a darkness at the edge of my vision, like a slow whirlpool in my heart.

In the early morning, before my wife arrives to take me home, I lift one more round of weights with Pedro. When I'm done we step out of the weight room and into the gym. Lara, one of the anorexics, has been allowed to exercise again. Before coming to the facility she was a ballerina. She'll be leaving in a few days, she has told me. The gym's single window lets in a shower of warm yellow light. Illuminated, Lara dances and leaps, and suddenly I don't want to leave. I just want to stand and delight in the beauty of her movements, which means I'm ready to go.

# Rendered Mute

TERESA BLANKMEYER BURKE

This is how to render a deaf girl mute.

Take One: I am chatting with a hard-of-hearing physician following a professional meeting. The conversation swerves from bioethics to personal lives, and I am asked whether I have children. Upon my affirmative answer, the doc inquires whether they are my biological children. When I reply, "Yes," his response shakes me to the core: I am incredibly selfish for bearing my biological children without knowing whether they would inherit my disability.

Take Two: I am dining with a childless-by-choice Ivy-League-trained hard-of-hearing educator, who tells me that deaf and hard-of-hearing parents who decide to bear biological children are cruel, abusive, and self-centered for not thinking of what a terrible life their children will have with a disabled parent.

I respond to these admonishments as a classic good girl; I sit there, silent, listening to their view of my decision to become a biological mother. That these professionals know what it is like to be deaf or hard of hearing is not lost on me. That we have reached different conclusions about the worth of our lives is lost on them.

A philosopher by temperament as well as by training, I consider their remarks. Was I a bad person for thinking that a deaf life was not so terrible? That, if my child happened to be deaf, then surely I might be able to manage this? That deaf ways of being in the world can be joyful and sublime? Had I committed the cardinal sin of

31

motherhood by saddling my children with a terrible burden from birth—that of having a disabled mother?

It is only now, as I write this essay, that I wonder if the difficulty I had in finding an obstetrician willing to go unmasked during labor and delivery was a response to my disability. I interviewed almost a dozen, but not a one was willing to let me lipread as I birthed. Was this a medical sort of shunning? If I were audacious enough to become pregnant, then I ought to shut up and comply with standard medical practice, even if it meant I would not understand what was being said.

But I knew that I would need to communicate during labor and delivery. I *wanted* to be able to understand any instruction or encouragement given to me. I *wanted* to be an active participant. After all, this was my body giving birth! All I needed was to be able to see the doctor's lips. Was this too much to ask for?

Fast-forward six years. I am a graduate student who has brought my nine-month-old daughter for a well-baby checkup at the university teaching hospital. My university does not provide medical insurance as part of the graduate student funding package, and I am one of many brown mothers in the clinic, but the only deaf one. The medical student who initially examines my daughter makes a comment. I miss it and ask the student to repeat what she has said. Upon my informing the medical student of my hearing loss, the tone of the entire visit changes. My daughter's medical exam is interrupted as the medical student shifts her attention to me. I am given a lecture on birth control and how to avoid becoming pregnant again, since we got lucky this time, but my next child might not be so lucky.

I am not only nonplussed but struck by the irony of "hearing" this from a dark-skinned woman of color who has undoubtedly experienced her own share of discrimination based on physical characteristics. I think about the kinds of things our children inherit from us. Things like a love of literature or an appreciation of nature.

Things like a distaste for cilantro and the ability to discriminate subtle gradations of color. Things like the family academic lineage and a people's history of persecution that my child of Jewish heritage inherited from his father. Things like a dimpled smile and a family history bound up with slavery and genocide that my child of African and Native American heritage inherited from her father. Things like compassion for people who have a different way of being in the world.

Before bearing my biological children I thought about the prejudices they might face—discrimination deeply rooted in historical fact, but also in the experiences of their able-bodied fathers. I did not consider the cruelty of bringing a child into a world where she or he would be highly likely to experience discrimination. I was not dissuaded by the taunts I had experienced as a child myself for having a mother of Arab American heritage.

But defying social discrimination is the province of good girls. Burdening innocent children with disability—whether their own or that of their mother—is the mark of an egregiously bad girl.

"How so?" I wonder.

Is there a threshold against which potential disabled mothers ought to measure their desire to become biological mothers against the harm their children might experience? And if there is such a threshold, are the harms of social discrimination related to disability unique? Or are these just a piece of the harm-continuum we consider when bringing any child into the world?

"But wait!" you interject. Social discrimination is different from physical disability!

True, that.

To have a body that doesn't fit into a world designed for a narrow range of bodies is frustrating. Dismaying, even. To have a body that experiences physical pain offers up a different kind of calculus from the one I performed when deciding to be a biological mother. Assuming that discrimination experienced by a deaf child (or any child of a deaf mother) is sufficient to forgo procreating is an act of medical prejudice. Leaping into biological motherhood, not knowing whether your child will be deaf or hearing, not believing your disability will harm your child, not knowing what the future will bring—well, this couldn't possibly be an act of love, could it?

This is how to render a deaf mother fierce.

# Jamie's Place

MICHAEL BÉRUBÉ

When Jamie was in his tween years, not long after we moved to the town of State College in Pennsylvania from Champaign, Illinois, I was asked to serve on the board of the local chapter of The Arc—formerly known as the Association of Retarded Citizens. (Nobody misses the "retarded" part, but I wish we could still say "citizens": it would underscore the point that Americans with intellectual disabilities are still citizens, with legitimate claims on the body politic.)

One of my tasks as a member of the board was to review the monthly reports from the group homes. These group homes seemed to be good places, but because they housed people with intellectual disabilities—like Jamie, who has Down syndrome—alongside people with psychiatric conditions, from time to time the living conditions would become unpleasant or even unmanageable. I was advised by my fellow board members that if I wanted to consider this option for Jamie in his adult years, I should probably start the wheels rolling when he turned fourteen. I decided not to do that.

I did not make that decision lightly, and I did not make it alone. My wife Janet heartily agreed, and for a while we imagined that, when Jamie was no longer in school, we would hire an au pair for him. And what, I wondered, might Jamie have in mind?

One night I asked him. "Have you ever thought," I said, "about where you might like to live when you are a grownup and a big man?"

"Mmm," Jamie said, nodding. "An apartment with a pool."

"You mean," I replied, knowing that the eleven-year-old Jamie sometimes spoke in sentence fragments, "you would want a pool in your apartment?"

"No!" he said, sensibly. "In the apartment *building*."

Very well then: that seemed plausible. I mean, the building sounded plausible. Jamie's plans, not so much. At that point in his life he really couldn't be left alone for half an hour; he was only just beginning to learn how to use the microwave, to shower, and to dress himself. Independent living seemed a very long way off.

A year or two later I asked him again. "Jamie, when you grow up, do you still want to live in your own apartment?"

Jamie seemed puzzled. "What?"

"You remember saying that when you are grown up, you would like to live by yourself in an apartment?"

Jamie modulated from puzzlement to alarm. He turned to me and exclaimed: "I don't want to be divorced!"

I stifled a laugh, because this was serious business. "No, no, sweetie, a divorce is when a husband and a wife stop being married. You would not be divorced. You would just live on your own—independently."

Wide-eyed, Jamie put a hand on my forearm. "I want to stay with you!"

Very well then: *that* seemed plausible. In fact it seemed like the most plausible option from every angle. (Though it dodged the question of where Jamie would live when we were no longer here, should he survive us.) So I made him a promise.

"Jamie, you can always, always stay with us," I said. "We love you so much and you will always be our son. We will never kick you out of the house! You can always have your room and all your things. But if you ever change your mind, we can talk again, okay?"

"I'll stay with you," he repeated, adding: "We have no other options" —a phrase he likes, and uses often, usually when he does not want to change his routine. So we left it there for a few more years.

With adolescence came puberty, and with high school came crushes on girls. Jamie and I have agreed—as we explain in the opening pages of *Life as Jamie Knows It* (2016) —that his emotional life is private, and that he and his father will not write or talk about his various crushes, then or now. Besides, the specific crushes are not the important thing. The important thing is that he had them.

So at some point I revisited the independent-living question. "Jamie," I said when he was either sixteen going on seventeen or seventeen going on eighteen, "you know how you said you always want to live with us."

"Mmm hmm."

"And, like I said last time, you can always live with us. But sometimes I wonder, as you get older, whether sometimes you would like a little privacy. You know, not just your own bedroom but maybe a little place of your own, right near us. Like if we changed the garage"—which is really a rickety storage shed, totally inadequate for a car, let alone a human—"into a Jamie House just for you?"

"Michael! That is impossible!" That is also what he said when I asked him if he ever had dreams about flying, so I assured him that although it was hard to imagine—and would certainly be prohibitively expensive—it was actually possible. Not plausible, not right now, but definitely more possible than flying.

By this point in his life Jamie understood not only the concepts of "public" and "private" with regard to standards of bodily propriety and bodily display (having learned to his surprise that the distinction can rest on the few inches of space between a locker room and a hallway), but also the quotidian procedures by which one washes oneself, dresses oneself, and makes oneself breakfast by reheating pizza, naan, Szechuan beef, fish tacos, or chicken tikka masala in the microwave. (Jamie will eat anything for breakfast except breakfast foods.)

Janet and I found that we could leave him to his own devices for an hour at a time, and one New Year's Eve, when Jamie did not want to go to a local party but we did, we managed to extend that alone-in-the-house time by another thirty minutes. Leaving at 11:30, we told him we would be back by 1 a.m.; and sure enough, at 1:00:00.00 of the new year (Jamie is nothing if not literal-minded—and punctual), we got a call on our cellphones. "Where are you?" he asked Janet. "Pulling into the driveway," she replied.

And did I mention that by this point in his life Jamie had learned how to use a cellphone?

When Jamie turned eighteen he became eligible for Supplemental Security Income (ssi), a program run by the U.S. Social Security Administration for the benefit of adults with disabilities. But he cannot accrue more than $2,000 in assets, and in 2011 he raked in $1,000 at work (recycling four hours a day—in the middle of a heat wave!—five days a week for five weeks, at $10.50 per hour) and another $500 or $600 in gift checks for his high-school graduation. So I put off the ssi application for a while. And then it took me another while longer to figure out how to get him a functional debit card. But by the time he was nineteen he could buy himself whatever he wanted—usually DVDs, Magic: The Gathering cards, and lunch.

Lunch was a surprise. One day I picked him up after he had worked from 11 a.m. to 3 p.m. volunteering at Discovery Space, the local children's science museum in downtown State College. "Should we get some lunch?" I asked. "I already did," Jamie replied. I was nonplussed. "You had lunch? At Discovery Space?"

"No, at Cozy Thai. I saw your colleagues, Jeff and Rich."

"You went to Cozy Thai by yourself?" I could imagine Jamie getting himself a sandwich from Subway or Jersey Mike's. But though

Cozy Thai was only a block away from the museum, I could not, at that point, imagine him taking himself to a sit-down restaurant with waitstaff and cloth napkins.

"And did you eat with Jeff and Rich?"

"No, by myself."

"And you paid for your meal by yourself?"

"Mmm hmm."

"Wow, that is so cool, Jamie." Jamie was clearly pleased. "Did you leave a tip?"

Jamie stiffened. "Shoot."

Tipping is so strange. I have read more criticisms of the practice than I can count—from restaurant owners and waitstaff alike. But it is standard practice in the U.S., and I didn't want Jamie to get a reputation in local restaurants as the disabled guy who doesn't tip.

Happily, Jamie is a quick study, and he soon mastered the minor but important life skill of taking himself out to restaurants for lunch and tipping. Though I also learned, by checking his bank account online, that he sometimes managed to rack up $35 bills at India Pavilion, his favorite restaurant (three or four blocks from Discovery Space), by adding special naan orders to the standard $8.95 lunch buffet and tipping very big.

On Wednesdays—which I began to call his Independence Days—he and I would get to the Pennsylvania State University campus (where I teach) around noon, and I would not see him again until 8 p.m., as he navigated his various appointments (music lesson), hangings-out at the Hub (the student center), and travels downtown. He had long since come to terms with the fact that he cannot drive a car and had become capable of getting himself around on municipal buses (for which he keeps a stash of tokens) and Penn State shuttles (which are free).

In the first chapter of *Life as Jamie Knows It*, I tell the story of the day in 2011 when Jamie came up to me and Janet in Central Park and asked: "Can I live independently?" What he meant, as I managed to intuit, was that he wanted to take the subway by himself to visit his cousin Trevor, who lives on the Upper West Side and has a very mild disability (he can travel independently and hold down a gopher job in a law firm). Janet and I said no, on the grounds that he very possibly could take himself on the 1 train from Columbus Circle to 103rd Street but would have no idea how to get from the 103rd Street station to Trevor's apartment. ("True," Jamie acknowledged, soberly.) But the following year he and Trevor took themselves to a Yankee game, then out for a sushi dinner at 11 p.m., then got themselves to New Haven on Metro North for a family gathering the next day. He and Trevor have since taken Amtrak—and, in 2015, Megabus—to visit an aunt and uncle in Boston.

Yet even as Jamie's independent living skills expanded to cover meals and travel, his plans for lodging remained the same: *I want to stay with you.* For four years, from 2009 to 2013, he took part in a program called LifeLink, in which people with intellectual disabilities shared an apartment for a week at a time, with the supervision of a 24/7 "life coach." He loved LifeLink—and, after our initial trepidation, Janet and I learned to like having a week to ourselves here and there—but he aged out of it at twenty-two. Since then his unstructured time alone has largely consisted of YouTube and videos in his basement lair, with an occasional break for playing my drums.

In the mid-1990s we had been introduced to the Camphill villages for adults with intellectual disabilities, but we didn't think of them as a serious option until recently, when I learned that a friend from grade school has a brother who lives in Camphill Village Kimberton Hills, 170 miles from State College. (That friend also told me how to get Jamie a nondriver's ID card in Pennsylvania; another friend from sixth grade now works for Social Security and helped me with Jamie's SSI forms. Such were the surprising benefits of joining Facebook and going to the fortieth reunion of my sixth-grade class.)

We visited Kimberton Hills a few years ago, but Jamie was emphatically not interested—and we noted with dismay that most of the residents were in their forties and fifties. The cost would be about $50,000 per year, and we could visit Jamie any time and even take him back home for as long as we wanted. The group homes near us, by contrast, are too restrictive for our use; none of us wants Jamie to live someplace where he can't join us on our various travels, which just happen to be his favorite thing in the world (yes, his favorite thing in the world is the world). So where does that leave us?

One half-chapter of *Life as Jamie Knows It* tells the story of Jamie's search for meaningful, fulfilling employment. This is, I think, the next great civil rights struggle for people with intellectual disabilities: access to the best jobs they can plausibly perform, perhaps with the support of mentors and job coaches—and financial incentives for employers. Under the Workforce Innovation and Opportunity Act (WIOA), signed into law by President Barack Obama in 2014, sheltered workshops for people with intellectual disabilities will be gradually phased out, along with their sub-minimum-wage exemption from the Fair Labor Standards Act of 1938. Jamie works in one of those workshops three days a week, earning about $1.90 an hour; he also volunteers at Discovery Space and at a local animal-rescue shelter; and he works at the Penn State University Press every Friday from 9 a.m. to 1 p.m., doing various cataloguing and inventory-maintenance tasks that draw on his intellectual strengths—his memory and his ability to think in lists.

But in the course of telling that story I had to take a step back—not only to remark that, in many places around the globe, an hourly wage of $1.90 would constitute a serious raise, but also to question what we mean by "meaningful, fulfilling employment." How many people are so fortunate as to have this thing in their lives? I am. Janet is. But we are not representative of all humans everywhere—or of all conscious entities, for that matter. I am thinking of the movie

*2001: A Space Odyssey* (1968), in which HAL tells a BBC interviewer: "I am putting myself to the fullest possible use, which is all, I think, that any conscious entity can ever hope to do." How many of us can say that? How many of us have settled instead for good-enough jobs that don't fully engage our talents and interests, but allow us to pay the rent and entertain ourselves from time to time? And how many of us yearn for one of those merely good-enough jobs, and would be perfectly willing to leave the "meaningful and fulfilling" criterion for some other aspect of our lives—a sport, a hobby, a church, or family and friends?

In writing about Jamie's desires for independence, I need to take another step back. This step, though, is even more uneasy. The disability rights movement in the United States, from its origins in the Bay Area in the 1960s, has always been about greater autonomy for people with disabilities: access to schools, to jobs, to buildings, to public space, to political participation. And this is why laws such as the Americans with Disabilities Act of 1990 and WIOA pass Congress with such bipartisan support—yes, even WIOA, passed at a time when nothing can get through Congress with bipartisan support. Liberals and Democrats support these laws because they expand the social welfare state and bend the arc of the moral universe toward justice; conservatives and Republicans like them because they promise to help people with disabilities become less dependent on support from the social welfare state. No one seems unduly flustered by the conundrum that we all need a great deal of help in order to become more independent.

There is a similar contradiction operating in the disability community. I try to capture it in one sentence: individual autonomy is indispensable as an ideal—and totally inadequate.

The "indispensable" part is easy to understand. It is woven into the fabric of U.S. life, from the Declaration of Independence to the legends of self-made men (almost always men) to the laments about twenty-something college graduates living in their parents' basements. More profoundly, it subtends our deepest hopes and fears about our bodies and minds: we want to remain in possession of our faculties, we want to make our own decisions, we want to be able to clothe and clean ourselves, we want to be able to travel freely and with minimal assistance (though, of course, with massive assistance in the forms of transportation vehicles and vast construction projects). We want to *live independently.*

But as the philosopher Eva Feder Kittay has been arguing for the past few decades, all the emphasis on autonomy—not just in U.S. life but in social-contract theory since John Locke—obscures our profound *interdependence* as a species. That interdependence is impossible not to acknowledge at the bookends of our lifetimes, as the very young and very old are obviously dependent on caregivers for their very existence, not to mention the maintenance of their routine bodily functions. But the rest of the time—for that hopefully long stretch between the Age of Pampers and the Age of Depends—we delude ourselves into thinking that we live independently.

And yet the desire to live independently is no delusion at all. Your desire for a little privacy, your desire to decide what to eat for dinner, your desire to visit your cousin—none of this can be dismissed as so much false bourgeois-liberal-individualist consciousness. Fulfilling these desires might very well, for many of our fellow humans, make the difference between a fulfilling and an unfulfilling life.

Late in the summer of 2016 we received a surprise email from the founder of a local outfit called Taproot Kitchen. Taproot is a farm-to-table operation in which people with intellectual disabilities learn to garden and cook—and, from time to time, cater events in the area. Jamie had been involved with Taproot for more than a year and had been delighted by the tasks of making pierogis, stuffed peppers, and (especially) Indian food.

Taproot was founded to address the problem of what happens when young adults with intellectual disabilities suddenly find themselves isolated and underemployed. "We address a problem shared by many young adults with ID who, upon turning 21, leave high school and lose their major systems of support," the Taproot website explains. "Job searches are frequently unsuccessful, and even when work is found (through the laudable efforts of agencies and job coaches), it can be unfulfilling."

Unfulfilling! Do tell. Taproot does: "Dishwashing, janitorial labor, and sheltered workshop piecework do not lead to the kind of flourishing that we know is possible for members of this community." Dishwashing, janitorial labor, and sheltered workshop piecework: that pretty much sums up Jamie's adventures with work life, except for his volunteer stints and his Friday mornings at Penn State Press. Now he also has Taproot once a week.

But this email wasn't about food. It was about lodging: a neighbor with a rental property next door to Taproot's headquarters (in a place called "the Meetinghouse on Atherton") was willing to sell the house to . . . well, to whom, exactly?

Some of the Taproot families began to meet. Could we collectively afford to buy a house and pay off the mortgage by renting it to our own adult children, who would use their SSI payments for a room in the house? At least two of those adult children were ready, willing, and (we hope) able to live in such a place permanently, with some supervision, and some were willing to give it a try for a month at a time. Jamie was reluctant at first, until I reminded him that right now all he had was his basement lair.

"Michael!" he objected. "We have no other options."

"Jamie," I replied, "this is another option. That's exactly what it is. Now you might have another option—living four blocks away from us for a month now and then."

A month seems too long to him, since he has known only week-long LifeLink respites from living with his parents. We suspect, however, that if this Taproot House becomes a real thing, he will quickly discover how pleasant it can be to live with one's friends, away from one's parents, for an entire month.

It is a daunting enterprise: four families have to form a limited liability corporation. We have to secure a mortgage at a rate we can afford. We have to spruce up the place (right now, it is a student rental, with all that implies) and work out a schedule of who lives where when. And then we have to find out if our kids-who-are-no-longer-kids can actually live together, living independently.

We did not see this coming. But I take heart in the fact that The Arc itself started, in 1950, as a grassroots parents' group—people coming together to try to address (and redress) the lack of social supports for people with intellectual disabilities. If this Taproot House works, it could serve as an alternative model to group homes and villages such as Camphill.

We have a lot of work to do to make that happen—Jamie, his friends, and all their parents. But for now, at least, we know one thing: we no longer have *no other options*.

Postscript: as of December 2016, the plans for Taproot House fell through. But we now have an LLC and may very well try again. . . .

# A Day in the Grammar of Disease

SONYA HUBER

If pain is a language, I have the accent on my tongue. I do not yet dream in pain, but a three-year immersion has stripped my skeleton's previous fluency. Now I am a child in this land without good parking spaces.

(10:30) Today my husband and I talked about my calcified hip and aching hands, the awkwardness of a threesome with pain. We parked outside my therapist's office, claimed the flowered couch, and spoke about those ball-and-socket hips: so essential for knocking socks. The words came small, with squinting, like picking lice. A hundred geese cursed and laughed from the glinting marsh beyond the open window.

The therapist, who emails me pictures of her baby goats, asked me to describe the pain as a number. They never ask the pain's name, which could be Fucker or Bunny. Then: Do you think you *are* the pain? I crunched my forehead to agonize in Venn diagrams: Am I coterminous with my disease? Overlapping?

It appeared that sex runways would have to be reconfigured, sex flight patterns remapped. The therapist smiled with optimism about the daunting industrial project of transferring a teenager's habit onto this irritable bag of Tinker Toys.

My body thinks you have rheumatoid arthritis.

This morning, (9:08?) pre-sex-talk, I saw a friend's picture on

Facebook: dyed jet hair, three-quarter profile, sharp lips in a punk-rock smile as she held the drumsticks aloft.

Later (11:45) I parked alongside the yellow-orange brick library and remembered the gold-tinged image. I winced: *Be careful not to hurt your wrists and shoulders with all that banging.* I saw in my mind a skeleton drummer, x-rayed with thick knots of danger.

*No, wait—that's me. Not her. She's fine.*

What grammar of disease operates beneath the surface of my skin and mind? As I called up the image, I reanimated Jenny with my own chemicals, crafted a tiny diseased punk-rock hazard. My body makes little bodies like itself.

I found Susan Sontag's *Illness as Metaphor* in the stacks; it was about cancer and TB, and I felt ashamed to be complaining, grateful to have the language of lifespan.

I am neither well nor doomed. Sometimes I watch your soft bodies not in pain and can't remember. I push forward, each day of appointments a wager.


(12:30) The afternoon brought a kitchen-table meeting about assignments and syllabi along with an ache like rung metal. In two hours the January clouds had seeped into my joints in a diagonal drift from the west. I tasted a pressure system change: the flavors sharp or dull, the directions inward or out, pulsing like a Northern Lights I had mindlessly devoured.

Synovial fluid in my joints is inflamed in an autoimmune festival, my own personal Burning Woman, a conflagration semi-controlled with drugs but without cure.

One colleague, a rock climber with enviable forearms and shoulders, sat across from me and talked Native American literature. I was distracted by the roaring of his body's utter silence, astounded as he angled fingers or turned a palm: he seemed to feel no pain, nor did he bargain with his skeleton. I wanted to interrupt the syllabi talk to ask if he hurt anywhere, but I did not.

I am new at this; such ideas still run like a secret world underneath this one. I am at a child's level of pain-chatter. Later, perhaps, I will learn to constitute and imagine a range of bodies inside me as a child learns to imagine minds unlike her own. Maybe I will not always have to ask: Can I show you mine, can I see yours?

(3:00) A final hot-chocolate cafe meeting, free wifi and essay-talk, the writing itself a bliss of disembodied mind-union, but then I had pushed it too far.

(4:45) I pulled on E into a gas station and shut off the car with a premonition like a migraine aura: it's cresting. It wants more room. Freeze.

I closed my eyes to see it, big and stupid. The attention this morning made it bolder. My pain stretched out and preened like a stuffed lion with a Farrah Fawcett mane, proud and full of itself: *Ruffle my head.* How could I hate something so mute? Goddamn floppy aimless pain, unsightly as my pilled and grayed stuffed animals from childhood, those transitional objects so close to us they seem to have our faces, our first containers for love and for loss.

# Marked

WILLIAM BRADLEY

"These tattoos provide a very positive tool in the treatment of cancer. During treatment they are necessary so the radiation therapist can precisely pinpoint the area needing treatment. After treatment they provide a history of the patient's treatment areas to future healthcare providers."
—John T. Gwozdz MD

"The body never lies."
—Martha Graham, American dancer and choreographer

For most of my life I have tended to go along without giving my body much conscious thought beyond the necessities of nourishment, excretion, and libido. It's really only when something is wrong—head congestion, leg cramp, shortness of breath due to the occasional panic attack—that I really think of my body. Even then, it's usually to think of it as something separate from me, something impeding my efforts to focus on what I want or need to be focused on.

As I enter middle age, though, I find that I've been thinking about my body more frequently. I never used to have allergies, for example, but now take Claritin at least once a day in the spring. Riding a bicycle—which was, for the longest time, my preferred method of transportation—now results in more fatigue than it used to. Not too very long ago, while lying on the couch with my head in my wife's lap while watching a movie, I suffered a back spasm that caused me to bolt upright and cross my arms in front of myself. She grabbed for the phone, thinking I was having a heart attack.

So I've been considering my body, and spending more time looking at it in the mornings before getting into the shower. I used to avoid doing this—as a young man, it was bad for my self-image to acknowledge the lack of muscle tone and—at various times—either scrawniness or beer-bloated heaviness of my upper body. But if I must be an old man—and apparently that's my fate—I feel obligated to look at myself and honestly deal with what I see.

As a nonfiction writer I'm most struck by the way my body can be read as a narrative of illness and injury. My oldest markings appear on the right-hand side of my body and tell the story of foolish accidents from childhood. In my right hip there is a small grayish-blue dot that used to be bigger but hasn't quite faded away. This is graphite from the tip of a pencil, jammed into my side while I was shooting a free throw during a school ground basketball game. I had forgotten that the pencil was in my pocket, and when I fell forward after putting all of my strength into the shot the pencil jabbed its way through the fabric of the shorts I was wearing and into my side. The injury must have been pretty severe—I remember going to the family doctor over it but not the emergency room. The memory has faded as surely as the wound has healed, but there's still that tiny dot.

There's also the hypertrophic scar just below my right elbow from the time I took the steepest hill in our neighborhood on my ten-speed, only to discover that the brakes didn't work quite as well as I needed them to in order to attempt such a feat. I went careening, ass over handlebars, into my neighbors' mailbox, knocking it down and messing up my bike's chain in the process. Luckily the neighbors were on vacation. To this day I doubt they know why their mailbox mysteriously "fell down." Though I suspected that I needed stitches for the deep cut in my arm, I just went home and put a big band-aid on it. I didn't want to get into trouble for taking out the neighbor's mailbox, after all.

The stories told by these scars seem kind of quaint, maybe even silly, in hindsight. At the time I'm sure I thought I had experienced great pain, but that was nothing compared to the tales the scars on my left could tell you.

The first and most obvious scar would be the one on my neck, which is actually three different scars from three different lymph node biopsies. I was diagnosed with cancer—Hodgkin's Disease— three times between the ages of twenty-one and twenty-four. These indentations that line my neck tell at least part of the story of those early adulthood years—hours spent kneeling in front of the toilet; the baseball hat that filled with my own shed hair in one afternoon; the lonely, terror-filled nights that eventually turned into exhausted mornings.

I have a smaller biopsy scar inside my right thigh, near my groin. This biopsy was done several years later, after a routine scan suggested I had a mass growing there. It turned out to be a mistake, but I have this small line there to remind me of the time that we thought my cancer had not only come back but had moved south.

I don't tend to notice these markings very often—they're simply a part of that body that, as I mentioned before, I tend not to think about. I'm not sure that most people who see them even notice them—nobody has ever asked. But people do tend to ask about the dots on my chest, splitting me right down the middle, when they see me without a shirt on. This doesn't happen too often as I get older and spend less time at swimming pools or water parks, but every girlfriend I've had since 2000 has, at some point, rested her head against my bare shoulder and pointed to one, asking, "What are these?" They look like freckles, only blue.

I'd always wanted a tattoo, but I've never been able to come up with a design that really expresses something important to me. I know that some people memorialize dead loved ones by inscribing their names on their skin, but I don't really have a dead loved one who I can honestly say meant so much to me that it would justify such a permanent reminder. An ex-girlfriend has the name of her two kids on her leg. That seems cool, but I don't have kids, I have cats. Getting a cat's name tattooed on one's body just seems ridiculous. One friend of mine—a professor of religion and very devout Christian—has the Greek words for "sin" and "grace" tattooed on his upper arm. That's a cool tattoo—personally important, but also rather scholarly. I'd like a tattoo like that, but all that comes to mind for me and my life are quotes by essayists. "Que sais-je?" "A writer is always selling somebody out." "As a writing man, or secretary, I have always felt charged with the safekeeping of all unexpected items of worldly and unworldly enchantment, as though I might be held personally responsible if even a small one were to be lost." But these feel more pretentious than genuinely expressive of my own personality or interests—although I must admit that the last one, written by E. B. White in "The Ring of Time," is sort of tempting. I have a feeling it would be a good conversation starter if I could unbutton my shirt at the hotel bar at the next academic conference to display that emblazoned across my chest.

So, no artistic, intellectual, or spiritual tattoo for me. But there are the blue dots. These were administered by a medical technician with a needle in February of 2000, when I was diagnosed with cancer for the third and—so far, at least—final time. Chemotherapy—both conventional and more aggressive—had failed to destroy my malignancy, so the decision was made that I should be treated with radiation. As we all know, radiation can be very effective at curing cancers, but also effective at causing cancers as well. For this reason doctors are careful about pointing the radiation beam directly and specifically at the malignant mass. To help calibrate their radiation machine they draw targets on the patient's body—for me those targets were tiny blue dots that go down my chest. My tattoos.

These little dots are not quite as explicitly spiritual as the religion professor's markings or as emotionally resonant as my ex-girlfriend's kids' names, but, I have to say, they matter to me. When I do happen to notice them, or when I do have to explain them, they call to mind all sorts of important things. They remind me of my mortality, which can be depressing but also inspiring—the knowledge that we don't have much time is an admonishment not to waste any.

More than that, though, they remind me of the absolute worst months of my life. I spent eight weeks getting treatments that caused me to vomit and the skin on my chest and back to burn and crack, seeping blood and pus. I had no family nearby at that point, and though I had many good friends who tried to help me, they were also living their lives while I—for the only time in my life—was thinking seriously about ending mine. I spent my days eating Wheat Thins and drinking Hawaiian Punch—nothing else appealed to my tumultuous stomach or inflamed throat. I sat around listening to Warren Zevon's version of Steve Winwood's "Back in the High Life Again," which was the saddest song I knew.

Why on earth, you might ask, would I want to be reminded of such a time? Perhaps for the same reason that my friend the Christian displays his faith on his skin or my ex-girlfriend the single mom has her kids on hers: Gratitude. Appreciation. It's been twelve years since I finished these treatments. As my health returned I vowed to never forget, to try to be a better person. But in the decade-plus that's transpired since then I have largely failed in those endeavors. I still lose my temper in traffic. I still forget to clean the cat's litter box despite promising my wife I will do it. I still have inconsiderate or selfish moments that disappoint, frustrate, and anger others. I'm not a monster, and I never was. But I can do better.

My tattoos—these blue dots down my chest that mark me as someone who has suffered, held onto his life, and promised himself that he would make that life count for something—remind me to do just that: better. Better than the self-centered person I know

I can be. Better than the lazy guy who shuts his office door and screws around on Facebook when he is supposed to be writing. Better than the short-tempered professor who sometimes feels personally insulted when his students fail an assignment. Better than the husband who unintentionally breaks his promises. Better than I am. The blue dots—like the other markings on my body— ultimately remind me of my own frailty and the need to live a life that I won't regret once it's over. These markings tell the story of my life. What's more, they remind me of the story's moral.

# 750 Words about Cancer

REBECCA HOUSEL

The ceiling creaks with every step. My family moves in clandestine patterns while I type at the computer in my red room below. The room is red for a reason, not just because I enjoy the color, though I do. The red is for passion, the kind of passion that can take a person to the extremes of joy and pain. I've been marked by both, and so paint my writing room red to remind me.

I seek the shrouded truth of Vedanta, the light of God in Christianity, the *sechel*, or reason, in Judaism, and the compassionate wisdom of Buddhism. All keys to the universe, just not mine. For a cancer patient there is no single key. How can there be? The universe is a large, complex place with many white-coated gods in sterile hospitals. Mine is a polytheistic world.

I have survived three cancer diagnoses in the last fifteen years, two brain tumors and melanoma. I'm thirty-three. Is there sense in sensibility? Is there brevity in wit? And what about the soul? Lots of questions, very few answers—that's something you get used to. You have to.

There are a great many "have-to's" when you face cancer. You don't want to have your skull drilled full of holes, then listen to doctors play connect-the-dots with a surgical saw and lift out your skull, exposing the fragile gray matter beneath. You don't want to be awake with a valium drip for the seventeen-hour surgery. You don't want to recognize in hour ten that you cannot move the left side of your body in panic and fear, and have an anesthesiologist named Surriel tell you to not be upset because you are going to sleep now. You don't want any of those things, but it doesn't matter what you want. You have to.

You have to face weeks in a rehabilitation hospital with nurses who disguise bullying with care. You have to go on to endure nine months of intensive chemotherapy where you lose ninety pounds, your balance, and your feelings . . . about everything. You have to consider the unthinkable: What will happen to my family if I die? What will happen to the $60,000 in student loans? Will my husband have to repay that if I die? Will my son grow up to be a good man? Will my husband find a new wife? Will anyone remember that I used to sit in a red room and write? Lots of questions. No answers.

I've made a discovery though, now being an expert on questions without answers. The question of why is always irrelevant. The only true question is *why not*. Why not? Why not die? Why not get sick? Why not get well? Why not travel to Australia? Why not live every moment to the very fullest? Why not. Not why.

The language is important. You predict the future with your words. Coelho's conspiring universe will help, too. You're like an alchemist trying to turn lapis exillis into gold. But there is no holy grail—it's a stone called moldavite, found in Moldavia.

The words you avoid are statistics and numbers. They deal in absolutes, and the universe is nothing more than string. Wave-like particles entangling with stationary particles . . . and then anything is possible, at least at the subatomic level. But isn't that where cancer starts?

There are one hundred and twenty varieties of brain tumors. Brain cancer is the third leading cause of cancer death. If you live in Australia, melanoma is the number one cause of cancer death. Over 190,000 people will be diagnosed with brain tumors in the United States in 2006. It's good to avoid this kind of language. Better to use the more fluid language of creativity.

We are not diagnosed with a deadly disease, we are merely *inter-*

*rupted*, as if in the middle of an engaging phone conversation, and then a child tugs at the hem of your blouse to ask an absurd question that has no answer; the question is being asked purely to distract you from the current call so you may pay more attention to the child. That is it. That is cancer.

You don't believe my words, my language? Maybe you don't want to believe. Belief can be suspended to let truth peek in under your skull and into your gray matter, the surgical saw still buzzing in your ear. Why? No, no . . . it's why not.

# The Power of a Handshake

HUGH SILK

I offer a simple enough gesture—a handshake. I have been told that my shake is weak and does not denote confidence, a wet-fish kind of shake. I am not concerned with how I convey power or strength, as my confidence brews deeper than my handshake.

But in this clinical setting, correctional health, the handshake is evaluated differently. I am offering it to an inmate even though we were instructed repeatedly during our orientation to avoid shaking hands with inmates. He looks up at me in astonishment as we briefly join hands.

Inmates are very careful not to come in contact with staff as this can result in disciplinary action. As I walk down the hallway, inmates will move to the side to let me pass and to be careful that our sleeves do not touch by mistake, which can be misconstrued as an act of aggression.

Some have downplayed the handshake in the medical setting for other reasons. With the transmission of infections on the rise, studies have shown that a fist bump may be a wiser choice for physicians with patients. There is certainly a place for the fist bump, but can we realistically train all patients to embrace it? And what will we lose with the omission of the handshake?

A wise old sage I worked with in medical school, who was a product of the generation where the physical exam was everything, would take each patient's hand and make at least ten observations from that handshake. How was their strength, their temperature, their ability to coordinate a handshake, etc.? Additionally, he explained how that simple gesture showed respect, initiated physical contact in a nonintrusive manner, and set a tone of partnership and friendliness. Bates and DeGowin could not have said it better!

Not long ago a retired warden came to speak to our medical team to be sure we were being mindful of the rules. On occasion a staff member has crossed a professional line, resulting in a breach of security. She was on message to remind us to be careful, to be cautious, and to be professional. However, she felt it was okay to shake hands. She told us: The handshake is a controlled act initiated by the provider and therefore will not be misconstrued; it can simply say I care but don't plan on taking advantage of that caring. It also conveys respect.

Medical care can never seriously be offered without a foundation in mutual respect. All too often that respect unfortunately flows only in one direction—towards the doctor. My best moments with patients are when they can feel I am interested in them, when I am complimenting them on their efforts and outcomes. Respect is a potent motivational tool. I learn so much when I just stop and listen. Every person has a story to tell.

And so here I am sitting with a man who has cancer. He is very aware of his options and has decided not to take the medical treatments that he sees as having too many potential side effects and too many potential shortcomings. He is choosing not to engage in false hope, and I find his reasoning sound. He clearly has done his homework, listened well, consulted with family (including medical types), and is confident in his decision. The conversation is not an easy one. I explain how I will care for him here, as I would care for someone in the community or my own family member.

I explain that there are limits to what we can get approved, but I will push for all the options at our disposal for maintaining his quality of life. I will see that his pain meds are appropriately adjusted, that he has an extra pillow (a big deal in a prison setting), and that

I will pay attention to the little things that we think will make a meaningful difference for him.

A family medicine colleague and friend of mine from Maine, David Loxterkamp, often paraphrases a thought from those who have come before us: we should be judged by the care we offer to the least of our patients. The words haunt me as I navigate care for the prisoners. Am I measuring up?

We stand to conclude the visit and shake hands for the second time today. This time his look of astonishment has changed to a look of admiration.

"Thanks for listening and for understanding. Nice explanations, doc."

We are eye-to-eye for a moment. The embrace is firmer now and we are both offering more through this symbolic contact. Today I feel I have measured up. Tomorrow we shall see.

At a recent national medical conference Eric Topol announced that the stethoscope was obsolete. Another low-tech tool that connects us to patients—gone. Let's hope the handshake stays with us as long as we are called upon to join with patients in a profession founded on caring.

# Submerged

TENLEY LOZANO

At the Mexican border, the rusty brown corrugated metal fence behind me, I pose for a picture at the southern terminus of the Pacific Crest Trail with Elu, my service dog. I plan to hike the Southern California portion of the trail in sections, starting with day trips and working our way up to backcountry camping. From where I stand in Southern California, the trail spans 2,650 miles, through deserts, over mountains, and into the wilderness before reaching the Canadian border in Washington, but I'm not thinking about the places the trail will take me; I'm stuck in the places I've been.

Over a year has passed since I've been in the ocean. It's been fourteen months since I've jumped into a pool. Sixteen months since I've worn SCUBA gear for my last operational dive in the coast guard, diving on an oil rig in Ventura. This might not sound like a long time to be out of the water, but for much of the last ten years I seldom went a week without swimming, diving, sailing, rowing, fishing, or living on a ship at sea.

When I left the coast guard I lost a part of my identity. I don't want to be in the water anymore.

A year before Elu and I will begin hiking the PCT, I'm sitting by the edge of a community center pool. I smell chlorine and, for an instant, forget where I am. I remember the feeling of tanks on my back, the struggle to hold onto my gear as an instructor rips it from my body, the sting of skinned knees and elbows on the concrete bottom, hands gripping straps that tether me to life-support equipment, a blow to my midsection that knocks air from my body.

I look at the edge of the pool, release my breath, unclench my fists, and will my neck muscles to release. I'm not in diver training anymore, haven't been for years, but my body doesn't always know that. I remember hanging onto the concrete edge, body and gear submerged up to my chin, the instructor—a chief in the coast guard—asking, "Do you know what happened there, Barna?"

"I didn't hold onto my gear tight enough, Chief."

"That's right, Barna. That's why I punched you. Don't make me do it again."

I recall telling my dive buddy, a man twice my size and a lieutenant in the navy, what the chief had told me. He was shocked and said, "He *punched* you?" I didn't think the hit was anything unusual until I saw his reaction. The punch itself didn't bother me so much as who it came from, a man that I will potentially deploy with as a coast guard diver, someone who I need to trust has my best interests in mind. I justify that he's enforcing a higher standard upon me because I'm a Coastie but know that it's likely that he's treating me differently because I'm a woman. I try not to think about what it might mean that this chief punched me underwater on a breath-hold specifically because I'll never fit in "The Brotherhood."

Sitting on the side of the community center pool, I put on goggles. I slip into the water and begin swimming laps, feeling the cool liquid on my skin and focusing on the timing of limbs and breathing. The movement helps me shake off anxiety. Flashes repeat in my mind, and I try to figure out why they bother me so much. Why does the smell of chlorine cause my body to lock up? Why do I feel amped for a fight? Later I will read that MRIS have shown that when people suffering from PTSD experience a flashback, part of their brain recognizes where they really are, but most of the brain experiences the memory as if the person is living it in real time.

After my workout, walking through the parking lot to my car, another unwanted memory resurfaces. I'm standing in a different parking lot by a different pool and a man is standing in front of me. He is tall and thin, looking down on me with dark eyes and black hair slicked back in a pompadour. Chief O'Donnell lays the ground rules for our working relationship, saying, "You will not speak when I am speaking. You will do whatever you are told, without question. You will not disagree with me or argue. You may be an officer, but I am a diver. Your rank doesn't matter because you don't know anything."

I want to argue, but he cuts me off, raises his voice: "As a female officer, you must never curse or tell dirty jokes, and must always be reserved." As he lectures me, I picture a 1950s housewife in a pretty pink dress with frilly apron, high heels, and a brass Mk V Surface Supplied dive helmet turning wrenches underwater. I want to roll my eyes, but if I show disrespect he will make me pay. "You will have to do dirty jobs, but that doesn't mean you can't be a lady at the same time." My throat tightens with anger and frustration.

Shaking off the memory, I am alone in the community center parking lot, no longer an officer, no longer in the coast guard, but still I want to punch Chief O'Donnell in the face. I want to know what would have happened if I had done something, anything, differently. If I had been more forceful, more persuasive, more aggressive, would he have treated me differently?

Just a few months after leaving the military I have mixed feelings about many of my experiences at the unit—fond memories of surfing or working out with junior enlisted divers that are tainted by the presence of the men who refused to work with me because I was female or because I was an officer. Every positive experience was subverted by a lecture afterwards.

Chief O'Donnell retired years ago. I separated from the coast guard in January of 2014, but my mind keeps reviewing these moments, trying to fit the pieces together. I run the scenarios and find flaws in my reactions, faults in my leadership, my willingness to please backfiring. Looking for patterns, I add situation after situation to the list of experiences that I wish I could forget and can't help but relive. Driving home from the pool, I feel like I'm being pulled deep underwater into the past, as if I'm holding a heavy weight and sinking fast.

"I am so sorry, Elu. I didn't think it would be this hot. Oh, nugget. Drink some more water," I say as I hold the collapsible water bowl out to my dog. Later I will ration our water, pouring three ounces at a time into her bowl, then drinking what she doesn't finish, ignoring the slight taste of dirt in the drool water. But for now I let her have as much as she wants.

We're at mile 64 of the Pacific Crest Trail and Elu is lying under the shade of a creosote bush, her short blond fur dusted with dark red soil as I rest on the dirt path next to her. We started the hike at dawn twelve miles back where the trail passed a road, and we'll be picked up tomorrow when we reach the next paved road. I'm hiding from the sun beneath pants, a long-sleeved hooded shirt, a hat, and sunglasses. It's 3 p.m., and I'm dismayed that I underestimated the desert heat and miscalculated how much water we would need on our first overnight trip. I tried to balance our hydration needs with the weight of the pack but failed.

A gallon of fresh water weighs eight pounds, and we began the day with almost three gallons of water. This twenty-six-mile stretch of trail doesn't have any creeks, water tanks, or spigots; there isn't anywhere to refill our water jugs, and we have to carry everything we need for the weekend. This is my first solo backpacking trip, so it's the first time that I have to pack all of my own water, Elu's water, my sleeping pad, sleeping bag, our tent, and our food. I don't even know if I can fit more water into the pack, but I'm feeling a tightness across my forehead that signals the beginning of a dehydration headache and wishing for sunset to hurry up and get here.

Elu wears her own pack, which has her kibble and high-calorie dog treats. She also carries trail booties and Musher's Secret paw wax, to protect the pads of her paws over miles of rocky terrain and coarse granite sand. Stuffed into one of her pack's pouches is a trowel in a Ziploc bag for digging catholes, my pStyle in another plastic bag (so I can pee standing up and keep my boots dry), and a red pouch holding her compressed sleeping pad.

As soon as the temperature began creeping into the eighties that morning, Elu's pace began to slow from our usual two miles per hour and I removed her pack, attaching it to the top of mine. By that point we had already consumed a gallon of water, so the added weight of her small pack wasn't overwhelming. I felt grateful for all of the hours I'd worn dive gear with a forty-five-pound steel tank strapped to my back and lead weights in the buoyancy vest's pockets. At least now my gear fits snugly, unlike the men's medium-sized equipment I wore as a coast guard diver.

Now I'm not worried about weight; instead I'm worried about Elu cooling down. "I shouldn't have brought you here," I say to her quietly, listening closely for her breathing to slow from its frantic pace. I tell Elu that it's just too hot for her. I promise to be more careful, announcing that we're done with overnights in the desert until it cools off. Most through-hikers, determined to walk the entire stretch of the PCT in one go came through this area two months previous. They had to make it through both the Sonoran Desert and the Mojave Desert to the north before the summer heat became oppressive.

I grew up in Virginia near the foothills of the Blue Ridge Mountains and wanted to hike the Appalachian Trail since I was a high school student. When the military took me west to Seattle and then San Diego, I was awestruck by the towering mountain ranges and the stark deserts that were so dramatically different from every-thing I'd known. My goal transformed into backpacking the PCT.

Elu's rhythmic breathing begins to slow and I relax, leaning into my pack that sits on the dirt trail, propped up by its fullness. I close my eyes and feel the warmth of the sun through my layered clothing. Listening to the buzzing of an insect circling my head, I stay still as a rock and look toward the erratic flying bug. It's a fly with multifaceted electric blue bubble eyes, its wings a vibrant blur. The creature quickly tires of me and darts towards Elu's nose. She appears asleep but doesn't hesitate to chomp her teeth at the fly, nearly biting a wing off and scaring it away. I chuckle to myself and shift my weight backwards, tipping the pack over on the trail.

I'm facing the sky now and I notice that it's a beautiful bright shade of blue, with big fluffy pure-white clouds being blown by the wind. I'm dehydrated and tired, and, despite all of the water I've been drinking, it's been too long since I peed. We're miles from what will become our backcountry campsite and even further from a road, but somehow I've found a moment of clarity. As Elu naps under the creosote bush, I realize I'm not anxious.

This is where I need to be.

I meet the resident psychiatrist at the Veterans Affairs clinic and shake her hand. She is young and pretty, with long dark hair tied neatly at the back of her neck. I learn that she is at the end of her year as a resident at the VA and that she will be transferring within the month.

I'm disappointed because I already like the woman; she seems genuinely dismayed that the system failed and I wasn't contacted for several months to complete my mental health evaluation and begin treatment. I trust her instinctively, but I promise myself not to like her too much, since I won't see her again. I separated from the military nearly a year and a half earlier, and since then I have been in a cycle of rejections and appeals to receive VA disability benefits.

She ushers me into a small office filled with a desk, computer, and three chairs, where I am thankful they've seated me facing the door. I'm better able to focus when I can see an exit route.

The resident psychiatrist runs through a list of initial evaluation questions in a kind voice as my service dog lies at my feet. I started training her a year ago, and I bring her to all of my VA appointments. She's a relaxed dog when she's on duty, and her ease calms me. I reach down and pet her soft ears as a painful memory threatens to overwhelm me. I explain how I feel when I'm in a crowded room, that I want to escape, and when I can't my body tenses up and I get panic attacks and migraines. I tell her how my dog helps, that she blocks people from standing too close, and she calms me down when I panic. It was tough for me to decide that I needed a service dog, since bringing my dog to public places makes my invisible disability obvious. But I feel more myself when she's beside me.

The woman asks if there is one main event that has caused my symptoms, if there is one time that I don't talk about, that seems bigger than the others. My throat tightens up, and I hold back unexpected tears as a memory overtakes me. A man is whispering something so that only I can hear, his body too close, the smell of beer on his breath, his hand on my shoulder, my skin crawling under his touch.

"He was one of my most trusted allies at the unit, but he was different when he drank. I tried to avoid his advances but I couldn't always do that, especially on deployments," I say. I try to figure out why this memory is so vivid, when nothing really happened beyond casual touches and his sexual advances.

He wasn't the only enlisted man to drunkenly tell me how beautiful and sexy I was, but the nature of our jobs required us to trust each other with our lives. When I was a surface supplied diver weighed down by my gear and hanging on a tether, I relied upon the people at my unit to physically pull my body up to the surface of the water. If I didn't feel safe with him at a group dinner, how could I believe he would have my back when I was underwater?

"Did you ever feel physically threatened? As if your life was in danger?" she asks.

My mind flits through a series of experiences and lands on one. I'm working underneath a coast guard ship, using a metal scraper to clean sea-grass off a propeller blade nearly as long as I am tall. I'm tethered to the surface by an umbilical that feeds me a steady supply of air. On my back is an emergency tank, but with this setup the tank is attached to the regulator on my full-face mask. I know that if my mask fails I will have to bail for the surface in order to breathe. My dive buddy, the same man who let me down again and again by hitting on me in front of our teammates, is out of sight scrubbing the other propeller.

A new unit policy dictates that all divers will rotate using the same equipment, not a specific set of gear fitted to each of our needs. The full-face mask that I normally wore leaked on almost every dive, but I'd gotten used to pressing my jaw into the bottom of the mask to keep it sealed. I had asked the chief in charge of equipment and the warrant officer before him to order the military-approved full-face mask that fit smaller faces without leaking, but they'd refused, saying, "No one receives special treatment around here. We can't afford to buy you fancy gear just because you like it better. Besides, you're a supervisor; you won't be in the water much anyway."

Working on the far side of the ship from the pier, I look down at the propeller blade and my mask shifts. Water flows into it and I press a hand to the front of the clear plastic, holding it to my forehead. The air flowing into my regulator sprays the water across my face. I can't see anything, and the noise of the air rushing over my ears overpowers the sound of voices coming through my earpieces. I spit water out and breathe in, filtering the spray by holding my tongue to the roof of my mouth. I taste salt and try to adjust the straps on my head, but they're already yanked down as tightly as possible.

I try to shift into a position where the mask won't leak, but no matter what direction I look water sprays across my face and I'm blinking frantically but can't see. I feel like someone has their thumb over a garden hose and is spraying me across the eyes. I don't think, just react, swimming blind. I'm spitting out seawater and moving under the stern of the ship by feel, making sure not to tangle my umbilical on anything, including my partner's line. I hear the comms unit sputtering, and I hold my breath but can't make out what they're saying. I reach the edge of the ship's hull and kick to the surface. I pull the mask away from my chin to let the water drain and breathe deeply, tears of relief mixing with the salt water as I fill my lungs with fresh air.

I'm frustrated and embarrassed that I couldn't finish the dive. Alone in my hotel room the night after the dive, I'll be angry when I realize that I almost died, and all because I wasn't given gear that fit properly. I pack the memory down tight and store it in the back of my mind. I hide it from myself, knowing that I can't let it affect my job as a dive officer.

A couple of months later, during a November deployment to Alaska, for the first time I will turn down the chance to dive. I'll glimpse beautiful and shockingly white sea anemones through the choppy surface of the clear blue water and pass up the opportunity to view that alien world up close because every cell of my body will tell me that it's too dangerous.

I'll try to talk myself into doing the dive, but my chest will tighten up and my breath shorten, and I'll feel like I might throw up. I'll quickly try to figure out why I'm so afraid of diving when I've never felt this way before. I don't know if I can take the spray of frigid water on my face and complete the pier inspection, so I'll act like I don't want to dive and let another take my spot. I'll try to ignore my shame at believing I can't do the job and rationalize that no one will respect me less for turning down a dive this one time. At that moment I will know that I've changed, but it will take me years to understand how much.

To the psychiatrist I say simply, "There were a couple times where my dive gear didn't fit and I almost passed out underwater, or I had to abort the dive because my gear malfunctioned." She types the note into my record.

I've been reading about PTSD and a prominent psychiatrist in the field, Bessel Van Der Kolk, who wrote about restoring the mind-body connection and reclaiming the emotional brain. Some of his research was focused on how yoga can help patients who lived through traumatic experiences. I regularly took yoga classes when I was in college and throughout Dive School, to unwind and balance the stress of never quite fitting in with the people around me. When I recently tried a session I was disappointed to discover that I couldn't relax because there were too many people in too tight a space. I can't focus on the movements when I don't know what is happening behind me. I quickly give up on yoga and hope backpacking with Elu will help me rewire my brain.

On the Pacific Crest Trail a jackrabbit nonchalantly hops in front of us, black oversized ears sticking straight up. Elu's body vibrates with excitement as she watches the tall grasses where the hare disappeared. "Leave it!" I say sternly and she whines, wanting to chase. "Aaaaye-looo!" I tell her in a singsong voice, and she sits down on the trail in front of me, tail wagging. "Let's go!" She springs to the end of the short leash, tugging at the waist strap of my backpack, where I've attached her lead. The fur on her back stands up and her right ear is perked, the left flopping and bouncing lazily as we hike.

I take in the details of the trail: rough salt-and-pepper sand under my boots made from crushed granite, short dark green greasewood, and the skeletons of long dead trees burnt in a wildfire years ago. I am learning to love the chaparral ecosystems of Southern California. Out here I feel again that my body is my own, as if I had been trapped inside a twisted simulacrum of myself, wanting to claw a way out of my skin. My past is always there, but now I'm not consumed by it.

Elu keeps me present on the trail. I watch her for signs of heat stress and am vigilant that if I am starting to lose concentration we need to stop for water and food. I talk out loud to her, telling stories and singing made-up songs, listening for the slurred speech and watching for the balance issues that precede a migraine. She tells me how she feels with her body language; ears perked, eyes alert, tongue lolling, lingering in the shade. Elu always lives in the moment and I'm learning from her. The constant movement allows me to stay focused. Elu relies on me, she believes that I know where I'm going and that we'll get there together. She's teaching me how to trust my instincts again, to follow impulses that I had to ignore in order to do my job.

Sometimes I don't say a word for miles and instead listen to the crunch of my boots on the sand, the rhythmic panting of my dog, the soft swoosh of my backpack as it shifts with every step. A black-chinned hummingbird's wings whirr in my ear as it investigates my brightly colored shirt. A cicada clicks a pattern that sounds eerily like a rattlesnake and I scan the ground in front of us for danger. I almost enjoy the feeling of blisters growing on my heels, and the weight of the pack on my waist and shoulders is comforting. I don't mind carrying Elu's water because she is excellent company. Alone on the trail with my dog I am happy, and the pain I feel is welcome because my body is mine again.

At the edge of the Anza Borrego Desert State Park, having walked the last seventeen miles without sight of another human, I suddenly feel the pull of the waves again and have a powerful urge to swim in the ocean.

# Where Do You Go from Alston Street?

KAT MOORE

Peanut hands me three white pills. She says it will help. She says *better than nothing*. We sit on the stoop outside her place. When we get high together inside her rundown apartment, splintered wood as walls, *don't drink the water*, no heat or air, and sometimes electricity, she says *this is my needle, don't set yours down, I got AIDS*.

The sun is out and the trees twist green around fallen-down rows of houses and fourplexes. Her brother, Junebug, behind us, a bottle of champagne in his hand, lives upstairs. He sells heroin but uses it, too, and smokes crack. When he smokes he thinks my glasses are microphones sending our conversations to cops. He thinks my bracelets are bugs. I stick out on Alston Street. I tell myself I can leave any time and never come back, unlike Peanut, stuck on Alston Street, hooking on corners, drowning in bathtubs when the AIDS virus has weakened her body and the dope is so strong.

Peanut says the pills are Clonidine. I hear Klonopin, an anti-anxiety med. Memphis is dry. No one has any dope, not even the Mexicans. All the dope tracks with nothing but sick junkies scratching fevers and picking at bone. *It will ease the sickness* she says. I pop them in my mouth. I get in my car and drive away from Alston, back to the white side of the city.

Clonidine is for blood pressure, and twenty minutes later mine bottoms out. I pull the car to the shoulder of the road. It's rush hour traffic and cars clog the expressway. My body slumps on a patch of grass glowing green in the sunshine. *Did I hide the needles and pipe?* Cars honk as I drift off to sleep. I dream I'm in my dad's pickup truck and we wind our way over gravel roads. Tires skid and kick rocks. My dad's window is rolled down and Luke the Drifter sings about *the bad girl who lives down the street.* I open my eyes and see paramedics. One snaps smelly salt under my nose. *What did you take?* And I'm singing again with my dad on an old country road. *Little girl,* he says.

Fluorescent lights flicker over my head. I'm on a gurney shoved to the side of a hallway. An IV sticks in the back of my hand, attached to a tube to hydrate me. My mouth is chalk. My lips stick together and I can't swallow. A nurse says *nothing to drink or eat.* I think they're punishing me because I'm a drug addict. A psych nurse appears and I say things like *rehab serenity house I need help* and she writes it down nodding. I don't know it, but my mom's in the waiting room waiting to see if they release me. But since I don't know this I tell the psych nurse I have nowhere to go. My car's impounded and it's late now, I'm not sure how late, but time has passed since I left Alston. The police found me on the side of the road and they called the ambulance and the ambulance brought me here. This is the MED. It's the poor people's hospital. That's what Elizabeth's mother called it, the beginning of the summer after ninth grade, right before my brother died. I had on my bathing suit and a towel around my waist. I asked for the phonebook. I wanted to check on my brother. He was at the MED. *Honey, he can't be there, that's the poor people's hospital.* And I dripped all over her carpet, *yes he is, he is dying of AIDS.*

I say I have to go to the bathroom. I pull the gown around me, *where are my clothes,* and I wheel the metal stand that holds the bag of saline that drips through a tube that is attached to the back of my hand. In the bathroom, I put my mouth to the faucet and drink up. My brother died in this hospital.

Plexiglass holding room. Nothing to break and use as a weapon on oneself or anyone. Little plastic recliners the slightest shade of purple are spread out in the small room, all facing the plastic mirror where nurses sit on the other side. I'm waiting for the psych nurse to tell them what to do with me. I'm back in my own clothes, my blue sundress with the cigarette hole in the right side and rust colored stains in a spot above the hem. Sometimes when I'm high I forget to wipe the blood off my arm and it smears across my dress and it's there permanently now. The dress is too big, *like a sack across you* my mom would say and tell me to never visit her at work in that dress again. It used to fit, it used to be pretty and clean. The room is cold and I ask for a blanket through the plastic but no one looks up at me.

Over to the side there's a bathroom with no door. I drink the water out of the sink and worry they mix soap in with the water because there are no soap dispensers and my mouth tastes all wrong.

Finally a student doctor visits me and takes me from the plastic room into a normal room with a real vase with fake flowers. I pretend to be dope sick but I'm not yet. Anxiety creeps back in and deep within me there's an opening and the pain's ready to travel up and howl through me. I need something to seal the crack before it spreads. He's young. He looks at me like I'm human. The lines of his cheeks soften and pity spreads across his face.

*When was your last fix?*
*Last night, around 10.*
*Last night? Four hours ago?*
*No, the night before. Before I last slept.*

*Okay.* He motions for the nurse. *Watch her,* he tells her. Then walks off down the hall and rounds the corner. I'm not sick, not yet. Peanut was right, the pills would keep it at bay, but moment by moment my body twists and tells me the sick will be here soon.

He comes back with a cup of water in his hands and waves off the nurse. He pulls a small package out of his pocket and pops two pills out the back of it. *Percocet should help.* I swallow them and want to kiss him. In a few moments warmth will glide through me, it won't be like heroin but it's better than clonidine.

The county mental hospital is where I end up for seventy-two hours of observation. Six Oh Three is what it's called. At Memphis Mental Health Institute, called MMHI for short, I'm in a room with three beds, one shower, and two other women. One's a spunky young thing who vibrates and rattles off about medication. *You need Haldol with lamictal and maybe thorazine.* I want methadone, meppergam, trazodone like the rehab I went to a few years earlier when I was still on my dad's insurance. Though once I did shoot up thorazine out of desperation. I also took acepromazen for dogs out of desperation—I curled around the toilet while my heart shook and my insides were static like an off-air TV channel.

My other roommate's nodded out in a wheelchair with a broken pelvis and pumped full of morphine. She stays that way all night, sometimes grumbling to someone in her nods. I toss and turn and my legs ache and my back hurts. I want to sink my teeth into her veins.

The medication line is long. One woman calls everyone Momma, including the men. This isn't like rehab. In rehab the men and women are mostly separated but in here we are all together. A heavyset woman rushes over to the momma caller and leans in close to her face. *I'm Brown Sugar and I'm your momma now.* The other lady cries.

I can smell Brown Sugar and it isn't sweet. It's days of refusing to bathe and change clothes. Later that day they drag Brown Sugar against her will into a room with a drain. Her clothes are stripped off and she's sprayed down with a hose.

While the line slowly moves, a man rolls around by himself in a wheelchair. His left foot touches the floor and propels him and the wheelchair forward. He's too big for the wheelchair. Almost seven feet tall, around fifty or maybe sixty or maybe only forty years old. It's hard to gauge age when life's been hard. He sings gospels in a deep guttural voice. My jumpy roommate sees me watching him, sees me swaying to his music. *That's Frank. He's a murderer, you know.*

I finally make it to the nurse's window. They hand me a huge horse pill. *Potassium.* I have trouble swallowing. Another pill. *Effexor.* At the MED I said the methadone clinic gave me Effexor. I hadn't taken Effexor or methadone in months. I don't know why I even mentioned it. I swallow the pill. The nurse tells me to wait. She comes out of the office with a syringe in her hand. *Ativan.* She injects it into my hip. It's not heroin and it's not mainlining but I will take it.

Ten minutes later it isn't so bad here.

We're shuffled from one fluorescent light-filled room to the next. Doctors we never see designate which groups we will be in. I'm in one about how to remember to take your medicine. I have never been diagnosed with anything that actually requires medicine, yet I have been given medicine because I'm a drug addict and no one seems to know how to help me. *Here's a pill. Swallow. It will make you feel better.* But it never did. Antidepressants turned me into a zombie. I don't even know what Effexor is for, but it makes me kind of sleepy and I like anything that slows me down and blurs the lines.

Brown Sugar's in this group. She eats an orange. Her nails dig into the rind and peel off the skin. The man in the white coat tells her that she can't have food outside of the cafeteria. She lifts a crescent moon of orange and crams it into her mouth then smiles with the guts of the fruit all over her teeth. The man next to her raises his hand and speaks before being acknowledged. He talks about leaving notes to remind himself to take his medicine. The man in the white coat tells Brown Sugar to throw away her orange, *there's no eating in the classrooms,* he says.

She says *I'm Brown Sugar.* This sends a ripple through the room. Voices chatter. Some laugh. The man in the white coat tries to regain control. I sit quietly. A little scared. I'm in a mental hospital against my will with others who are here against their wills but they, unlike me, have diagnoses like *bipolar with schizo-affective disorder, borderline personality*, and don't leave after three days.

The room buzzes. People are shouting. The man in the white coat raises his voice. The man next to Brown Sugar, the one who needs notes to remember his meds, snatches the rinds off the table and then grabs and pulls what's left of the orange out of her hands. He walks over to the door and tosses it all in the trash. He returns to his seat. Everyone shuts up. Brown Sugar says *damn.*

My mother drops off clothes and cigarettes for me. I'm happier about the smokes because no one here really wants to share. Smoke breaks are spaced out through the day. During those times we are led outside to a huge paved area with tables, benches, and basketball hoops which stay empty and cast shadows across the concrete. Ward Four West shares the area with us. They are a little bit crazier than my ward, Four East, but not nuts like on Five. I sit on the ground and lean back against a light pole. A tall thin man with curly brown hair pinches the filter of his cigarette. He talks to an older woman who nods and says *yes, yes, yes.*

He's having a party and he wants her to come. His house is out in the country somewhere or maybe Cordova which is a suburb but feels far away. His party will have beer and music, lots of music and dancing. The woman nods *yes, yes, yes.* I want to be invited to his party even if it's pretend, even if he doesn't know the right location. Outside of this place I don't have anyone besides my mom. Maybe Brendan but he has a girlfriend and he only likes me because I do drugs just like he does drugs but everyone knows how I do drugs so he keeps our friendship a secret. I had friends. Jenny and Tiffany I met in college before I dropped out but they moved to Japan. James was my friend until I repeatedly stood him up because I was off copping dope. Cherry is dating a guy, an artist who rarely drinks and never does drugs except pot but that doesn't really count. I try to bat my eyes at the guy with the pinched cigarette but he won't stop looking at the older woman with a double chin and receding hair. *There will be philosophy there, too,* he says. And she says *yes, yes, yes.*

My last Ativan shot kicks in and the man with curly hair becomes two men with curly hair but more like conjoined twins whose contours blur together. I look around the courtyard and everyone's doubled. I close my right eye and cup my right palm over it. With my left eye I scan the people sitting on benches and tables. All smoking. All folding into themselves and then unfolding again. I take off my glasses and do it again. I switch eyes. One of the guys from my ward sees me and says *and she ain't crazy, just a drug addict,* then laughs.

It's exercise time. We stand in the day room in our regular clothes. We always wear our regular clothes. I'm told it isn't so on other wards like Five, but that we are in Four East and it's the laid-back ward. I imagine skin and bones in faded blue scrubs and shuffling feet in slippers above our heads. A lady comes in the dayroom. She walks in circles around the dayroom, around the tables, the stiff sofa, and the plastic chairs. She tells us to fall in. We all follow her around the room. We walk in a circle for twenty minutes. She says *good job* and then leaves the room. This was our exercise time.

Growing up, I read books like *I Am the Cheese, The Catcher in the Rye,* and *One Flew Over the Cuckoo's Nest,* and I fell in love with the struggle of class and crazy (though Holden was rich and disillusioned, but I did not pick up on that then). I watched the old black-and-white film *The Snake Pit* starring Olivia de Havilland. I locked myself in my room and pretended to be in a mental asylum undergoing psychoanalysis and electroshock therapy. I also read *Junky* and *The Basketball Diaries* and watched the movies with the same names and pretended to be a heroin addict, burned bottoms of spoons and faux shot up with ink pens.

I call my mother to complain about the tedious conditions and to make sure she understands that I don't belong here. She says, *It's like those movies and books you love. You should be excited.*

The cafeteria looks like a school's cafeteria. A young black man stands in front of me in line. Every few seconds he says *Carlos tried to suck my dick. Fucking bitches and hoes.* I know what it's like to be fucked up because of things that happen to the body. The times when your body doesn't belong to you.

The guy behind me says *Damn, Carlos done fucked you up.*

The line inches forward and I hear it again, *Carlos tried to suck my dick. Fucking bitches and hoes.*

Once we get through the line I follow him and sit across from him. He's a pretty man, high cheekbones and delicate hands, light-skinned with blue eyes brighter than the sea. His hair is pulled back into tight braids.

*Hi.*
*Hi.*
*What is your name?*
*Rayvonne.*
*I'm Kitty. Short for Katherine.*

He sits and eats and stares like he is somewhere deep inside himself and he doesn't know how to get out. If I ask a question he answers it but offers nothing else.

*How old are you?*
*Twenty-three.*
*Me, too. Do you like it in here?*
*No.*
*Me, neither,* I say.

Then we sit quietly across from each other poking at the food on the plastic trays with our plastic forks. He drinks chocolate milk and I drink tea but really want a Coke, almost as bad as I want heroin. Rayvonne slugs back his milk and doesn't mention Carlos again.

Day three and I stand in line for meds, and when I finally get to the window I'm only handed potassium and Effexor, no nurse comes out with a syringe to poke in my hip. My seventy-two hours should be up. I tell the nurse I want to leave and she says it's up to my doctor. A doctor I have yet to see. She points to the double doors, the ones that lock and you have to be buzzed back in. She says *she's right outside those doors in her office, she'll let us know when it's time.*

*But I've never even met her.*
The nurse shrugs. *It really doesn't matter.*
*My stomach is upset,* I lie. *I'm still sick.*
*You can't have any more Ativan* she says, then offers me
    Pepto.

In the dayroom I sit on the edge of the off-white sofa and keep an eye to the hallway watching the double doors. My hands shake. My brain shakes. I'm thinking of ways to get out of here, which is really thinking of ways to get high. People mill around this room. Brown Sugar sings Whitney Houston's *Greatest Love of All* and the woman who calls everyone Momma holds a doll and dances. Frank roves around in his wheelchair shouting bible verses in a deep voice. One of my roommates sleeps in her wheelchair and the other one tells a woman I don't know about Haldol and how it makes her tongue stick to the roof of her mouth.

A man sits down next to me and introduces himself as Jerry. We have polite conversation. He's coherent. We talk about Memphis, about the weather, about the high schools we went to. He makes jokes about the other patients and I laugh. Then he turns his head to where no one is and says *I'm not talking to you. I done told you to hush up and let me talk. Hush up.* He pauses, waits for the air to respond, and then turns back to me. *Sorry about that, he's so rude.*

I'm discharged the next morning without ever seeing a doctor. The front desk, the gatekeepers of the main entrance, gives me a voucher for a cab. The cab driver can only take me to the address the hospital gave him. It's a long drive to my mom's. Down Poplar, near the homeless drop-in center, I see a man laid back on the grass; a forty-ounce beer in a paper bag leans against his thigh. I want to be him. I want to let go and leave it all behind and sleep on the grass with a forty-ounce and not have to worry where my next fix is from. Not have to worry about withdrawals or cars in impound lots and mothers who will get cars out of impound lots, mothers whose hearts get broken every day, mothers who kick you out at times and you worry where you'll sleep and if it'll be safe. I once heard a man say that the first time he slept in an abandoned building that he was scared but then eventually he got used to it, he adapted. I want to be there. All the way there where I don't have to worry anymore about being me because by that point surely the me I am now will be gone.

It's nightfall and I sit in Peanut's small apartment on her thread-bare burgundy couch. The electricity is on and the lamps shine and the TV, knobs as dials, hums images across the screen. I drag on my cigarette and flick ash toward the tray on her cluttered coffee table. I dip my syringe into my water glass, her glass is on the corner by her leg. She says *this is my needle, don't set yours down, I got AIDS.*

I tell Peanut *after you gave me those clonidine, I got sent to MMHI.*

She laughs but then says *why do you keep coming back here?*

And I say *because I am just like you* though I still don't believe it's true.

# Confession

DIANE KRAYNAK

The questions are unexpected.

"Have you ever robbed a bank?"

"No," I say.

"Have you ever killed anyone?"

"No."

"Okay then." Father Tom lays his hands on my head, says a prayer, and absolves me of my sins.

I'm in confession, and the priest and I have been talking for two hours. I chose to take this sacrament face to face and avoid the anonymous dim, smelly confessional booth with the scowling Angry Jesus picture that I remember from my youth. It's been over thirty years since my last confession and they call it "reconciliation" now. The luxury of this personal approach is the allowance of time. After reviewing my entire adult life Father Tom, a kindly septuagenarian, and I veered off into other philosophical topics. With nothing more to confess, he asked about robbery and murder. I assumed he was joking and I denied the claims.

"Thank you. I'm sorry I was here so long."

"Oh, no problem. If you want to talk more, just give me a call." With that, Father Tom escorts me out of the Jesuit parish rectory and into the late spring evening.

I drive home in silence. The sun slips behind the Smoky Mountains. I thought confession, an unburdening of the soul, would feel more cleansing. I don't feel particularly lightened. My hospital identification badge is still clipped to my dress. It lies heavy on my chest.

Have you ever killed anyone? The question unnerves me. I'm a nurse. I'm a healer. I'm supposed to help people. Uncomfortable memories suddenly surface: patients, colleagues, and situations I haven't thought about for years rush back.

I remember pushing my fingers into a baby's chest for twenty minutes, but none of the pressure would bring him back to life. I remember standing next to a little girl with a Do Not Resuscitate order, watching lines on her monitors flat-line. I remember the stunned grief of the mother who was told we weren't going to start dialysis on her son because his overall condition was too grave and the dialysis would be futile. There were others: too many children we couldn't save, too many parents we couldn't console.

By the time I reach home I've tallied up my failures. My boyfriend Scott calls later that night. "How was it?"

"Fine. He asked me if I've killed anyone."

"Well, you haven't."

"I'm a nurse. My patients die."

"But you didn't kill them."

I grasp at images and feelings, feebly articulating what I'm thinking. But the pictures are gauzy and my words are clumsy. "I don't know. How are we defining killing?"

Mirage dies a few weeks after my confession to Father Tom. Mirage is part of a herd of horses near my house. I ride one of his herdmates, Sundrop, and I consider Mirage to be one of my own. A majestic Tennessee walking horse, he is the alpha and at twenty-nine years old is still going strong except for a little arthritis. On a Tuesday morning Mirage slips in the pasture and can't get up. His leg is broken. The woman in charge of the horses that day brings the herd up late for their breakfast; she is busy with upcoming trail rides. The people running the barn don't do a head count. No one notices he is missing.

Four hours later a kayaker spots a black horse alone in the field, struggling to rise. He calls the barn. The vet arrives first. Mirage is dehydrated. He has baked in eighty-degree heat for four hours, suffering with a broken leg. He is put down immediately. His owner can't get there in time. She couldn't say good-bye.

Mirage's former owner is my riding instructor, and she erects a shrine in his stall at the barn. We lesson students bring things for the altar: pictures, his halter, his bit and bridle. The black toy horse I bought him for his birthday joins the offerings. We huddle together under the barn lights and share Mirage stories.

The woman we accuse of killing him cries when she sees us. We're silent in our grief and fury.

"I'm so sorry! I was so busy. It was an accident. I'm so sorry!" she wails repeatedly.

I'm uncomfortable watching her cry. Something in me stirs and I open my arms to her. She sags into them, sobbing harder. Hugging her, I feel like a traitor to Mirage, but the woman's pain seems genuine. My riding friends remain immobile during this exchange. I hope these are not crocodile tears.

I'm back at the rectory entrance waiting for the solid oak door to open. I trace the outline of the slate patio with my shoe. The door hinges creak. Father Tom appears at the threshold and ushers me back into the same moss-green room as before.

"You said I could come back if I wanted to talk." I resume my place on the cargo sofa.

Father Tom settles into his chair. "Of course. What's on your mind?"

"You asked me if I killed anyone."

He waits quietly.

"I'm not so sure I haven't."

"What do you mean?"

"It's not really a fair question to ask a health care provider. I'm a nurse. People die on me all the time. One Christmas our NICU lost seven babies in ten days, and five of those assignments were mine. I've turned off ventilators and unhooked IVs. I've done CPR on a baby but couldn't get the heart beating again. As a nurse practitioner I've been part of discussions where we decided to discontinue care or not get things started. I put my cat down because she only had months to live and I wanted her to die on my schedule before she got worse. Does any of this make me culpable of killing?"

Father Tom puts his palms together and places them over his lips. I tell him about Amadeo.

My boss calls me at home on a January evening. He's a physician but I call him Fred. He's a kind, quiet man and one of few words. "We have a new consult. NICU." "Okay. Do you need me to come in?"

"No, no. We can't do anything tonight. Just come to NICU in the morning."

"What is it?"

"Polycystic kidney. We don't know how bad but if it is, we need to plan for PD catheter. I'm arranging with the surgeons." He sighs.

"What's the baby's name?"

"Amadeo."

Amadeo's kidneys have cysts, bubbles of fluid that formed in his kidneys while he grew from an embryo to a baby. These fluid-filled cysts expanded, encroaching on the rest of the kidney, pushing the normal tissue out of the way and making the kidney bigger. Amadeo drew the unlucky straw of having cysts in both kidneys. His kidneys and lungs jockeyed for space in his tiny abdomen but the kidneys, being the heavyweight, won the fight and squished his lungs high into his upper chest. The lungs didn't have room to grow and thus didn't develop properly. Amadeo was born with kidneys too big and lungs too small.

There was a time in the not-so-distant past when these babies would die at birth because the lungs couldn't breathe, the kidneys wouldn't work, or both. Not breathing is an obvious cause of death, but without kidney function there is no way to urinate. Without urine excess fluid and toxins build up in the body. Potassium goes up. Blood pressure goes up. The heart beats faster trying to rid the body of the extra fluid but to no avail. The heart floods and the body drowns in a sea of toxic fluid. Exhausted, the heart gives up. Death comes shortly after. But not now. Now we can take out Amadeo's kidneys and start him on dialysis to give the lungs room to develop and do their job—breathe.

Since Fred is talking to the surgeons, I know the plan: dialysis. Through a combination of biology, chemistry, and physics, dialysis will work in place of his kidneys. First, a surgeon will place a flexible plastic tube in his abdomen. A nurse will infuse a special fluid of water, sugar, and electrolytes through that tube and into Amadeo's belly. The fluid will mix with his blood and this mixture will pass back and forth across his peritoneum, which acts like a membrane. Good things like blood and protein will stay in the body while waste products and extra water go out. He'll do this every day until he's big enough to be transplanted with a kidney, at least two years from now. Until then infection, poor growth, and death are among some of his constant threats. Amadeo has a long, rough, uphill, twisting road ahead of him.

This newborn intensive care unit is my old territory. This unit molded me into the nurse practitioner that I am today. These white walls, scuffed linoleum, and overhead lights cradled me as a nursing student. I chose to work here after graduation and I learned how to be a nurse among the rows of incubators and monitors. This NICU is where I observed my first delivery, performed my first CPR, witnessed my first death, administered my first postmortem care. I no longer work as a unit nurse here but my friends are still around.

"DK. You here for Amadeo?" My friend Bobbie catches me in the hallway. She is one of the nurse practitioners. She was my preceptor when I was a student and is one of the reasons I chose to work in the NICU.

"Yeah. Fred been in?"

"I haven't seen him. Baby's cute."

Bobbie leads me to Amadeo and we join Sue, another friend and Amadeo's outgoing night shift nurse. "Hi honey," she says, stifling a yawn.

"Hey."

Amadeo looks up at us. He's a tiny baby boy with chocolate eyes and raven curls. "You guys doing dialysis?" asks Sue.

"That's the plan."

"Glad I'm off for a few days."

Dialysis stresses everyone. The mere suggestion of it causes much hand-wringing. I know why the nurses are anxious. Fred and I are a new team together, just over two years. His predecessor didn't do much, if any, dialysis. With volume comes experience and with experience comes proficiency. We're going to do dialysis on a baby in a unit where there's been no volume, thus no experience and certainly no proficiency. I saw dialysis once when I worked in the unit, and it wasn't with the equipment we're going to use. This combination of a new modality and inexperience threatens everyone's confidence. They're fearful of failing; for if it doesn't work, new procedures will be sought and the line between helping and meddling blur, and his care could segue into needlessly prolonging life. They are worried he'll turn into a Science Project—the moniker for babies who languish on the altar of "because we can, we do."

Fred and I talk to Amadeo's mom. She's from my hometown. She has the same dark hair as her son. Fred walks her through the upcoming steps. Dialysis. Growth. Discharge. Transplant. We discuss the many obstacles to overcome, the labyrinth of complications that can happen. Mom is hopeful. Deep dimples accentuate her smile.

I go to the operating room for Amadeo's surgery. One surgeon, Dr. B, puts in the peritoneal dialysis catheter. Another surgeon, Dr. X, removes the kidneys. They are rust colored and lumpy and look like a bag of marbles. Both kidneys are thirteen centimeters long, over six and half inches. Normal newborn kidneys should be around two and half inches. Amadeo's evicted kidneys overfill the stainless-steel specimen bowl. We take turns staring at them, resisting the urge to pop the cysts like bubble wrap.

As surgery winds down Dr. F, the anesthesiologist, pulls back the sheet covering Amadeo's face. Amadeo is white. Too white. There is sudden activity at the front of the bed. Labs are drawn. Blood pressure is retaken. His hematocrit, a measure of red blood cells that carries oxygen through the blood, is 4—dangerously low. Without oxygen being able to get to his brain and organs, he will die. Everyone starts talking. The activity speeds up.

I call Fred from the OR. "His catheter is in. Kidneys are out. And his crit is 4."

"No. That can't be. His hemoglobin would be 1. That's not possible."

Dr. F is pushing blood into Amadeo, who is slowing pinking up.

"No, I think that's right. His kidneys were thirteen centimeters apiece. Apparently they had all his blood supply."

Jamie is the nurse taking care of him after the OR. I fill her in on what happened. "Was his crit really 4?"

"Yep. The kidneys are huge. I think Dr. X took pictures."

"When are we starting?" she says, referring to the dreaded dialysis.    "Twenty-four to seventy-two hours. Hopefully seventy-two. The longer we can wait and let the catheter incision heal, the better." We discuss what will give him a successful prognosis. I put my hand on her shoulder. "We'll be fine."

Our hope for Amadeo is not misplaced. The dialysis works. He's gaining weight. He's eating. He's doing well. By mid-February he's cleared this hospital hurdle. He's ready to go home. We will follow him in our outpatient clinic. I'm coordinating the last of his discharge plans when Bobbie calls from the NICU.

"Amadeo has a fever. We've already done a blood culture and the fluid culture is pending."

"We're on our way."

In healthy people fevers are useful. The high temperature helps the body fight infections by denaturing the viral or bacterial proteins. In compromised patients fevers are concerning. Compromised patients are targets for opportunistic infections—viruses, bacteria, fungi, all lying in wait like a mugger ready to assault an unsuspecting victim. Amadeo's age, his hospitalization, and his dialysis put him in the compromised category. His fever is worrisome.

Fred and I arrive at the bedside. Fred furrows his brow. Amadeo looks puny. His color is off and he's not as alert as he usually is. The fluid coming out of his belly is cloudy. It should be crystal clear. None of these are good signs. We get the confirmation soon enough: fungus has infected Amadeo's peritoneum. Fungal peritonitis can be fatal because we have to stop the peritoneal dialysis while we clear up the infection. We need an alternative treatment.

Amadeo's medical team confer together. We decide to try another form of dialysis, hemodialysis. A different surgeon removes Amadeo's belly catheter and places one in his neck. Through this catheter a hemodialysis machine will pump out his blood, push it through a filter to clean it, and then return it to him. This dialysis is most often used in adults, larger children, and teenagers. It's a daunting and dicey plan with risky complications: blood loss, infection, death.

We feel Amadeo is worth the risk and we reconvene at his side. Amadeo's fever has come down and he looks better. He stretches in his sleep. The hemodialysis nurses have arrived with the equipment, but they look worried. They are experienced dialysis nurses with adult patients, not kids, and certainly not newborns or infants. Through no fault of their own, no one here has dialyzed a baby with hemodialysis.

Fred sucks in his breath. The surgeon put in an Eight French catheter. It's too small. Catheters are thin tubes like straws. The wider the tube, the faster the fluid can travel. If the tube is too narrow, incredible pressure is required to keep the fluid moving, much like drinking a milkshake through a cocktail straw. An Eight French catheter is insufficient for hemodialysis. We need at least a Ten French catheter.

The dialysis nurses shift nervously and fiddle with the machine. The narrow catheter will likely not work but we have no choice. We have to do something.

"Let's get this going," Fred says.

We give up on hemodialysis the next day. The nurses can't keep the hemodialysis machine going. It needs to pump the blood fast but the catheter can't handle the pressure. The force needed to move the blood is destroying red blood cells and making the machine stop. It's straining Amadeo, the catheter, and the machine. We're going to hurt him if we keep this up.

We try continuous renal replacement therapy, another form of hemodialysis but with a slower blood speed. The dialysis nurses run into the same issue. The catheter is just too small. They start, stop, and tinker with the machine for a shift. We can't get this to work. Amadeo is getting sicker. His laboratory values are changing for the worse, he's getting puffy, and his blood pressure is going up. Nursing is getting agitated. We're on the precipice of hurting versus helping him. It's starting to feel like an experiment. Someone mentions "Science Project."

We give hemodialysis another try but the same problems persist. Dr. B is out of town and his colleagues refuse to attempt placement of a bigger catheter.

"Why?" I ask Fred.

"I don't know." He runs his hand through his hair. "They're not comfortable. They're worried it'll be too big and tear his vein."

"But if we don't do a bigger one, what do we do?"

Fred doesn't answer.

"If we don't do dialysis, he'll die. It can't get worse than that, right?"

Fred stays silent, staring at Amadeo.

"Can we do two Five's? We need a Ten French, right? A Five for venous and a Five for arterial? Will that work?"

"No. Not here. I suggested but they don't do that here."

Peritoneal dialysis isn't available to us yet. His peritoneal dialysis catheter was removed and we're still treating the fungus in his belly. Surgery won't operate on his abdomen while he's infected. We concur, as that would certainly make him sicker, but now we're out of options. There are no more tricks, no more work-arounds.

"So what do we do?"

Fred closes his eyes, massaging his forehead with his hand. "Nothing."

We stare at each other. We went from planning his discharge party to signing his death warrant. It's not supposed to be like this.

Fred and I meet with Mom on a dish-water gray Friday morning. We're at Amadeo's bedside. He's been moved to the back row, by the windows. White vinyl privacy screens surround him. Staff and nurses drift in and out to hold his hand and stroke his cheek. It's déjà vu. When I was a nurse here, I had a "Science Project" one spot down.

Mom understands the technical quandary we are in. She doesn't want him to suffer. She agrees to no further care. She is gracious as she accepts the plan.

The dialysis nurses pack up the machines. In the upcoming hours Amadeo's blood pressure will go up. His potassium will go up. He will lose consciousness. His heart will stop beating. The nurse taking care of him has tears in her eyes. Fred holds Amadeo's hand in his fingers. We can't stay. We have patients to see across town in our outpatient clinic.

"I need to say goodbye to him," I say. "I'll meet you over there."

"Okay."

It is my turn to hold Amadeo's fingers. He has plumped up since birth and inherited Mom's dimples. I try not to cry. Mom gives me a hug.

"Thank you. Thank you for doing all this."

"I've done nothing."

"You gave me six weeks with him."

"I'm so sorry. I'm just so sorry."

"You did everything you could."

Did I?

She squeezes my hand. Tears drip down my cheeks as I slip out of the unit doors. I sniff and weep my way across town. I'm late but I detour to 7–Eleven. I stagger into the convenience store, dazed among the familiar smells of linoleum, burnt coffee, hot dogs, and gas fumes. Coffee in hand, I queue in behind a dapper elderly black man chatting up the clerks.

He turns to me. "I'll get that."

"What?"

"I'll take care of that."

"Huh?"

"Your coffee's on me."

"Oh no, I couldn't."

"Really, no, it's my pleasure. You look like you need it," he says. "Please. It's on me."

I want to hug this old stranger with his gentle eyes, in his shiny brown suit, and smelling like Aqua Velvet. I want to tell him we just said good-bye to a baby—that with all our tricks, tools, and toys, we couldn't get a catheter or machine to work and keep him alive. I want to ask him why in twentieth-century America, right outside of our nation's capital, the power center of the world, we can't save this baby.

I croak out a thank you and flee.

Fred meets my eyes when I arrive. We move through clinic in silence, trying to be present to those in front of us, hoping they don't notice we're distracted. Their problems are important to them. We can't tell them about Amadeo and that today we think they have no problems.

Clinic is finally over and we're alone. Snow flurries wisp outside.

"You staying?" Fred asks me.

"I'm going to finish these notes."

He lingers in the doorway. "Okay. See you."

"Bye. See you Monday."

Years later Fred and I will be working in a large free-standing children's hospital in the Midwest. A baby with the same disease will be born. A surgeon will take out her kidneys and put in a peritoneal dialysis catheter. She will get fungal peritonitis. She will get a hemodialysis catheter. She will get hemodialysis six times a week for three months until we can do peritoneal dialysis again. She will live. She will be transplanted. She will thrive. I will look at Fred and say "This could have been Amadeo." He will shake his head sadly. The remorse lingers.

Father Tom shifts in his chair. The afternoon light sparkles on his white hair. Before he can respond I continue.

"I looked at the board on Monday—just to see if he was still alive by some miracle. His name wasn't there."

I tell him about Mirage. "I'm hugging this woman and I'm thinking 'you killed him' and then I think of Amadeo and think that I did the same thing.

"I know it's different but somehow, they remind me of each other. Mirage fell. He broke his leg. He would have been put down regardless of when they found him. But if that woman brought them up on time, maybe Mirage wouldn't have fallen. And if he did fall, if they did a head count, they would have found him and maybe he wouldn't have had to suffer for four hours. Mirage died because a woman failed to do her job. Amadeo died because we failed to do our job. When you asked if I had ever killed anyone, I thought of him. I know it's different but it seems the same."

Father Tom takes his time to answer. "It's more of a team failure, don't you think? You alone didn't do this. For Amadeo, the mother agreed to no further care. Isn't that what you said?"

"Yes. She did. On one hand it seems like we did all we could but on the other hand, it feels like giving up. I remember feeling like we worked hard, like we gave it a valiant effort. But we didn't have what we needed so we just stopped."

"Without any intervention, would he have died at birth?"

"Yes."

"Those other babies, were they following the natural course of their illness?"

"Yes."

"It's not the same, you know that, right?"

I stare absently out the window. I try to sort out the guilt I've taken on. "I don't know. We stopped care. We left him. I'm part of that 'We.'"

Father Tom pauses again before he speaks.

"I'm very sorry about Mirage."

"Thanks. I guess that's a team failure too. Other people at the barn could have noticed he was missing."

"Have you thought that you helped the family?"

"No. Not really."

We are quiet, absorbed in my story. Father Tom says a prayer. I head to the door.

"You're being too hard on yourself," he says.

"Maybe. It's still a provocative question to ask a health care provider. We all have blood on our hands."

I go to the barn before it closes for the night. The herd grazes in the pasture. I wonder if they avoid the spot where Mirage fell. My chest tightens. The question unsettles me. Have I killed anyone?

I approach the fence. Sundrop is a few yards away, golden in the fading light.

"Hey, sweet girl." I make kissy sounds to her. Sundrop lifts her head, pulling a weed up with her. Grass pokes out of the corners of her mouth. She locks her eyes with mine and swishes her tail.

# This Moment

ADRIANA PÁRAMO

This is it. This is the moment our lives crack wide open like a pomegranate and all its bloody bits spread long and wide.

One month before my daughter turns sixteen I stand by the hospital bed, look her in the eye, and ask why. She stares blankly at the ceiling, fidgets with the D-rings on her oversized cargo pants, while the social worker questions me about our family life. Where is her father? Is there violence at home? Any history of drug or alcohol use? Where did she get one hundred ibuprofen?

I ask her again. Why is life with me so unbearable? She rolls her eyes, turns her back, curls her fists into tight balls and faces the wall.

I wish I could do the same.

The nurse walks in to check on my daughter. I force a smile and a *thank you*, but she doesn't react. Maybe she thinks that the children of good mothers do not attempt suicide; don't rebel, don't spit fire, don't curl their hands into tight fists and turn their backs. Maybe she thinks that I drove my own child to the edge with my flaws, my ignorance. I want to defend myself, my daughter, us. But all I have is this moment. This iv drip. This wailing ambulance braking hard outside.

The social worker wants to know about home. Home, I repeat in my head. The word resonates with all its accommodating possibilities: noun, adverb, adjective, verb, but its linguistic elasticity gives me no comfort.

It occurs to me that if I tell the social worker how beautiful our home by the water is, with its balcony overlooking a lake, the cathedral ceilings and the vast backyard, everything would be fine. But the woman is impatient; she taps her pen on the clipboard, and the lovely feeling is gone.

My thoughts scatter, senselessly. What if this is happening because we live in the wrong house? What if we had bought the house in Auburndale instead of this one? It was a grand-looking old house that sat atop a hill overlooking Lake Ariana. It had Moorish archways and Mediterranean-looking windows; wooden floors that creaked and ceilings that slanted; two whimsical attics, a kitchen with a stucco counter, and a black furnace in the perfect corner. It also had asbestos, copper plumbing, and a moldy roof. Naturally we didn't buy it, but now I wonder if maybe a touch of mesothelioma would have kept us together; if disease would have made us more compassionate, more loving, better people. Maybe the asbestos and the mold would have glued the seams of our lives.

When I'm informed that she'll be put under suicide watch, I recite a mental litany: My love, the door is open and translucent for you to see inside me. I won't make demands, I won't judge, I won't speak. Just give me a sign, and I'll be weightless, patient, tender. Let's name that which we lost along the way. Let's bury the unnamed thing. Let's give this thing a name and punch it square in the throat. Let's sweep it under the rug. Let's fix this. Together. Let's. Do. Something.

They bring her into the room to say good-bye. The underwire in her bra has been removed, so have the shoe laces, her pink scrunchy, her belt, and the flaps of her baggy jeans. Her eyes beam with an anger so fresh and mean that it makes my whole body tremble. I'm supposed to say something reassuring, something magical, something important. I'm the mother. I'm expected to mend this broken child. But I can't.

She climbs slowly into the van. I wave, but she turns away.

I can't breathe. I need to be monitored too. Preferably next to her. Put us into solitary confinement together. Beat us and starve us and do not let up until I put her pieces back together. Until she is whole, finally or again. The van signals a right turn, slows down, then disappears around the corner, leaving me behind in the middle of the street on my knees. I stay there feeling a sharp rock under my left shin. And I cry. Not for my daughter over whom I have lost complete control, but for the manageable thing. This pain digging into my flesh. This thing with a name and a solution. This hurt that I can stop. This that I can fix.

# Sit Still and Uncover Your Eyes

ELIZABETH BRADY

The passageway of grief is lined with a thousand doors. I've read this description in a variety of places, not attributed to anyone in particular, but I like it. I often picture the long hallway ahead of me, light sneaking out from underneath the closed doors. In the early weeks after Mack's sudden death I would stand in this hallway unsure of what to do. But now I open the doors and walk in because I always find him there.

Our beloved son Mack died suddenly of sepsis on New Year's Eve 2012, two weeks shy of his ninth birthday. Our community of soccer, church, family, and friends gathered over the next few days—lifting my husband and me and our daughter and carrying us, for a time, as we all shared the horror of Mack's abrupt death.

But those times are pauses in life when we come together to honor passages: births, graduations, weddings, and death. Our loved ones come alongside us, but none of them can take on our grief any more than they can create a marriage for us. They must eventually go attend to their own lives, leaving us to face our agonizing new reality.

"There is no question of getting beyond it," Katherine Mansfield wrote in a 1920 letter in which she reflected on death. "The little boat enters the dark fearful gulf and our only cry is to escape—'put me on land again.' But it's useless. Nobody listens. The shadowy figure rows on. One ought to sit still and uncover one's eyes."

And what does it mean to sit still and uncover one's eyes? For me it has come to mean facing death and choosing life, sometimes several times a day. But it is not facing death as some abstract notion, it is facing Mack's death and choosing to continue to live and love him and our family.

One of the doors I open most frequently is Room 37 in Penn State Hershey Children's Hospital, where we arrived behind the Lifelink helicopter. The blood infection hit Mack like a bolt of lightning and overtook his kind heart in a matter of hours. His dad and I cared for his body one last time. We sat on either side of him. I swirled Mack's wild hair through my fingers with my left hand, and my right hand held Christian's hands in Mack's, resting on his chest over his Winnie the Pooh hospital gown. We sobbed over his body until our tears dried up.

"Your baby," Christian said to me through tears. "Your buddy," I said to him. And we stood up and held each other over Mack. And we still do.

It is in Room 37 that our dreams for Mack and his vibrant life, and the dreams he had for himself, were severed.

But it is also in Room 37 that I was struck silent by Mack's repose. I dabbed my tears and drank in his face, his long, dark eyelashes at rest on his cheeks and the right corner of his mouth turned up into a slight smile. It was a smile I knew well when he was bemused. What did you see? Who came for you? I have asked him many times. His smile speaks to the beyond, to the place where I believe I will join him upon my death.

In *Hour of Gold, Hour of Lead*, Anne Morrow Lindbergh wrote that part of the process is the growth of a new relationship with the dead. It is a hidden, quiet journey within and it requires me to sit still and keep the door to my own spirit open.

I am not afraid to walk into these rooms anymore because each time I allow myself to venture in I find Mack, whether in a dream, a memory that causes me to burst out in laughter or tears or even a nudge to buy or do something for someone he loves. I have learned to accept these moments of grace as the "flecks and nuggets of gold" in grief that Anne Lamott refers to in her book *Traveling Mercies.*

Mack's early, sudden death still takes my breath away. But, by facing the truth of his death and choosing to live and love him and one another, I am able to embrace my whole life with my eyes uncovered.

# Overtones

MEREDITH DAVIES HADAWAY

"Would you like some music?" the nurse asks her patient, while I stand with my harp in the doorway of his hospital room.

"It don't matter," says the boy.

All elbows and angles, he shifts in the sheets. Pain and fever have made him sweaty and bright. Hair the color of autumn soybeans sticks out from his temples in little peaks. He doesn't speak but slowly turns to face me, one arm braceleted in yellow that says *Fall Risk*.

I wheel the harp into the room, sit on a small folding stool I have carried with me, and begin to weave through a series of slow airs connected by improvisatory passages—"The Water Is Wide," "Farewell," "Welsh Home," "Eleanor Plunkett"—I play longer, sweeter, slower, hoping he will sleep. His eyes stay open but his feet stop jigging under mounds of white. On the tray between us I see the slight shiver of water in its cup.

The first time I played music for someone in medical distress, it was my husband who was dying of lung cancer in our living room. I had never heard of "therapeutic music" but had spent fourteen months at my husband's side through x-ray, bronchoscopy, biopsy, diagnosis, referrals, long commutes, chemotherapy, radiation, surgery, and recurrence. Now we were home, cut loose by the medical team at Johns Hopkins who had been our constant support while he was a poster boy for their protocol. When metastases turned up in his liver, they delivered the bad news and never returned another phone call. Large teaching hospitals are for the sick—not for the dying.

Now we returned to our rural, small-town facility, where the nurses knew my husband by name—some had been his students. They countered his fevers as best they could, spooned ice chips into his mouth, and kept his room as quiet as hospital machinery would allow. When word went out that his children had been called to his bedside, a queue formed outside his room of others who wanted one last chance to say good-bye. Though he had not been communicative for a month, he rose to the occasion, hearing the testimonials of love, nodding assent to requests for forgiveness, even offering a final quip to some of the friends and neighbors who came softly, one by one, into his room in the ICU. After a few hours the nurses threw everyone out and the silence resumed as his room took on an evening glow.

"Please let him die tonight," I thought, sitting beside him in the golden light. But I knew that would not happen because death resists our notions of perfection.

It was a week later, back at home, when his half-sleep of morphine ended suddenly. He had been too weak to turn himself, yet he leapt off the hospital bed we had placed in the window by the river. He was standing up, pointing a finger, saying one word over and over—"once."

The hospice nurse had warned me that the young, the strong, would sometimes struggle at the end, but this strength seemed superhuman and I was frightened. He was extremely agitated—even back in bed he twisted and shuddered. I called his local doctor, a longtime friend. It was Sunday—he was on the golf course. Our bottle of morphine drops was nearly empty and still my husband would not quiet. I reached the doctor's wife who persuaded our small-town druggist to open his store to get us more drops. But the wait was interminable and I was desperate.

In order to calm my own anxieties and with some vague notion it might help his, I placed a CD in the player—Eric Satie's "Gymnopedies." The slow, steady pulse and spare harmonies filled the room like a breathing presence. Within a few minutes my fear was gone and I felt a palpable peace settle around us. By my side, my husband's eyes closed and his breathing was slow but more regular. The agitation was replaced by utter repose. His facial muscles were relaxed but not slack. His arms lay gently at his side. He looked beautiful.

We breathed together in that space for what seemed a long time—though by now the minutes slipped by unnoticed. The music played on, thanks to the repeat button on the player—an otherworldly soundtrack for the breaths that now slowed to a pace I could not match. Long pauses. Longer pauses. Eventually only the strands of Satie's strange chords floated bodiless in the air around us.

Years later I'm wheeling my thirty-four-string Celtic harp across the parking lot of a nearby residential hospice facility. Partly because I want to "pay it forward" in honor of my husband and partly because I thought I could use a little healing myself, I have enrolled in the Music for Healing and Transition Program (MHTP) to become a Certified Music Practitioner (CMP). Despite an annoying profusion of acronyms, I chose the program with the most rigorous requirements: ninety hours of classroom instruction in healing modalities, science of sound, assessment of patient conditions, music theory; lengthy independent reading and study, on-site bedside experience at a large medical center, and the opportunity to gain experience in hospitals, nursing homes, and hospice environments, keeping detailed patient logs and working under the supervision of a trained advisor.

MHTP is one of several programs that offer training in "therapeutic music," which the literature describes as "live acoustic music, played or sung, specifically tailored to an individual patient's immediate need in order to bring music's intrinsic healing properties to the bedside." Similar programs have sprung up with the rise of complementary medicine, training musicians to offer comfort to those facing the myriad challenges found among the very young, the very old, the sick, and the dying.

The harp seems to be particularly effective for reducing pain and anxiety and inducing relaxation, so many therapeutic musicians are harpists, playing small folk harps better suited to the bedside than the large pedal harps seen in concert halls. The music tends to be fairly simple—easily digestible, based on folk or hymn tunes, chants, or improvisations in structures that vary with the desired effect. Often the session starts at fifty to seventy beats per minute, echoing a resting human heartbeat, and slows gradually to induce sleep or relaxation.

"Entrainment" is how we describe music's ability to change the physiological responses of those in the room, heartbeat slowing with the music's pulse, respiration matching the musical phrase. My role is to inhabit the shared space of the music with those in the room, be they conscious or unconscious, patient or family member. This differs from "entertainment," where the content of the music might dictate tempo and selection. For nursing home patients we try to play recognizable tunes, hoping familiarity will enhance a sense of identity and stability. For premature babies we play lullabies that sway in ¾ time, often in the higher registers more like a mother's voice. The music we play for those who are actively dying tends to be arrhythmic or very loosely metered, matching the patient's inhalations and exhalations rather than heartbeat. At the end of life the goal is to help the patient "let go," so we avoid the distraction of earthly melodies.

When I arrive at the hospice residence, the nurses ask if I might go immediately to the room of Mr. Q, a gentleman who is in distress. I can hear an alarm going off down the hall as he resists the restraints that are in place to keep him from falling—even louder, groaning interrupted by long strings of expletives.

"We're so sorry," the nurses say, as if the harp were too genteel an instrument to accompany such indignities.

"Not at all," I say, "this is exactly why I am here."

Mr. Q has thrown off his covers and I see that he is wearing only a diaper and that his body is covered with welts and scratch marks. A nurse sits beside him, trying to rub his back through a latex glove.

"Hush now, please. Just listen to the music," she says. Despite her efforts to soothe, he shouts and struggles.

I start the bass line vamp for a languid version of "The Water Is Wide" that is my go-to opener till I can assess the pulse of a space. But this time I don't move on from that four-measure intro. Something tells me to repeat the vamp, slow and steady, like a solid heartbeat. Over and over I let the deep notes ring at a tempo that seems to thicken with each repetition. Now Mr. Q is lying back, turning sideways toward the music. His eyes are closed. I let the bass line rock us both again and again with a regularity that would be monotonous if I couldn't feel and see that it was working. So we rock together, Mr. Q and I, in a slow, deep cradle of sound. Within five minutes he's asleep. The nurse has tucked the covers back around him. I have perfected the tiptoe departure, my harp attached to silent rubber wheels for just this purpose.

In the course of my six-month practicum I play for many hospice patients. Some distressed, most just resting. Some are alone, some surrounded by family members. Rarely do I leave a room where anyone is still awake. One son dropped off with his cell phone still in his hand in a chair where he had been holding a bedside vigil for his dying mother. As I turned to go, she roused enough to nod toward him and smile. Even at the end a mother is a mother and a son is a son.

The nursing home is a more challenging gig. The patients vary widely in their needs. Some, confined because of purely physical limitations, still have their wits about them. Others appear robust but suffer cognitive deficits and dementia. When I arrive for my first session, I sign in at the desk.

"We are so glad you are here," the attendant says.

"Because I've brought a harp?" I ask.

"Because the patients are restless—the Elvis impersonator didn't show." I look up from the clipboard—she's not kidding.

In contrast to the serenity of the hospice facility, the nursing home is bustling and noisy. My first assignment is to quiet a small group of patients gathered by the nursing station "trouble-makers," I am told, wheeled there so the nurses can keep an eye on them.

I start to play "The Water Is Wide," but an elderly gentleman interrupts—"Do you know 'Greensleeves'?" In general, we don't play requests, but I shift to "Greensleeves" in A minor and he settles back in his chair.

"Can you play 'Ave Maria'?" a frail woman asks. That one I cannot fake but I weave "Amazing Grace" into the mix and she seems satisfied.

"My brother says you look like a baby doll," another woman says, gesticulating toward a water cooler. "Oh, he's got his eye on you."

"Please be quiet," says the nurse. "This woman has a *gift* she wants to share with you."

Once I feel the music's pull, I try to keep it going, weaving one song into another to avoid any interruption that might break the spell. By the time I've been through "Greensleeves," "The Water Is Wide," and "Amazing Grace," the group is quiet, some watching my hands, some looking into their laps, one watching the water cooler. I play for fifteen minutes, winding down with a slow "Farewell."

"These are our rowdies," the nurse says, "especially at this time in the afternoon—and you've tamed them."

Well, they do appear subdued.

"I'll be in heaven soon," says the woman who asked for "Ave Maria." "There will be *real* music there."

"That made me sick," says the man who asked for "Greensleeves." "Every note carved a hole in my chest."

"Oh dear," I say, "I'm so sorry."

One tiny woman waves me over to her wheelchair and takes my hand. "Can you get a message to my family?" she asks. "They don't know I'm here."

The value of recorded music in nursing homes has been powerfully demonstrated by filmmaker Michael Rossato-Bennett in the documentary *Alive Inside*. The film follows Alzheimer's patients who receive iPods loaded with music from their earlier lives to show how many become engaged, communicative—even mobile—from simply listening.

Live music, played "prescriptively" at the bedside is believed to offer different benefits, in part because the tones that emanate from a musical instrument offer a range of frequencies known as overtones. Vibrations from the fundamental pitch join vibrations at a mathematically predictable series of resonant frequencies, engaging our neurocircuits across a broader spectrum to produce a richer auditory experience.

The more obvious significance of "live" vs. recorded music is the connection that occurs when another human is present, whether a nurse, a priest, a hospice volunteer, a loved one, or simply a stranger with a harp. Whatever vibrations emanate from the harp strings, they are part of a less-predictable set of overtones that is the emotional energy of another human presence, providing awareness—whether conscious, semiconscious, subliminal, or via some more mysterious means—that we are not alone in our struggle, in our illnesses, in our aging, in our various and even final transitions.

I have seen profoundly deaf patients respond to the music with a smile, a tapping of fingers on blankets. What do they hear? With impairment they might not make out the meandering melody of "The Water Is Wide," but they are moved by something larger than the limits of our hearing, something rich with overtones.

And who is to say which frequency is the "fundamental"? In the hospital room the boy who told me "It don't matter" tugs at his covers with the large, reddened hands of a farm worker and settles back into the pillow. Seated across from him, I pluck at strings with the small, waning fingers of a sixty-year-old woman.

"You should make a CD," he finally says, "so people know you're out there."

"I'm not out there," I say. "I'm here."

# The Way of the Spring

PATRICK DONNELLY

I believe I was infected with HIV about 1984; I tested positive in 1989 when I was 33 years old. In September of 2017 I'll turn 61.

In the decades since I was diagnosed, being infected with HIV has changed from an almost certain death sentence to a manageable chronic illness, but only in parts of the world where people have access to both general and specialized health care and insurance to pay for that care. What I would tell a person newly diagnosed with HIV today is that your life will change, and you will have to become a spiritual warrior on your own behalf, but you can have a fully realized life.

What I would tell a person without access to treatments is— well, I would say nothing: I would hang my head in shame and dismay. The fact that millions of people go without the treatments that have saved my life is a grievous injustice that I don't begin to understand.

Each person must make his or her own decision about living openly with HIV or not, because unfortunately—ridiculously, outrageously—in some places there is still a stigma attached to the diagnosis. From the beginning I chose to live openly, on the reasoning that it would expend a huge amount of energy to keep a secret as big as this one. I knew my energy would be better spent fighting to be well and to live my life, and I've never regretted this decision.

HIV affects each person differently, and each person differently at different times, as is of course true of other illnesses. I've often thought it was somewhat ironic and humorous on the universe's part to make mine a path of life-challenging illness, because I am not a person who is very good at being sick (if there is such a person). I've been known to go completely off the emotional deep end about having a cold that dragged on longer than I would prefer. Therefore it's fortunate—more than fortunate, damn lucky—that my life with HIV has been relatively easy. From 1989, when I was diagnosed, until 1994 I used a variety of alternative medical treatments, successfully for the most part. In 1994 I became quite ill with general malaise, low-grade fevers, and eventually the cancer Kaposi's sarcoma inside and outside my body, as well as two bouts with pneumocystis pneumonia (PCP). The latter two opportunistic infections killed many people during the early years of the AIDS epidemic; I was probably about a year or less from dying at that point. Today it frightens me to read the medical journal I kept in those days. Even to touch the book or walk near the shelf where I keep it inspires dread. Some researchers have suggested that receiving a diagnosis of life-threatening illness, or the onset of symptoms, can cause PTSD, and I have never doubted it.

But when I began antiretroviral therapy in 1996 (using the second, more effective generation of such drugs, which doctors were also much more skilled at prescribing), my immune system reconstituted itself quickly. Since then, though there's always some small-to-medium problem to manage, I've had a wonderful life, and am in many ways healthier than some people without HIV. Now, when I read that some relatively young person has died of HIV, I often wonder if some other factor (alcoholism, drug abuse, psychological factors, etc.) was to blame, stressing the immune system beyond its capability to adjust and recover. Even as I write this I have to admit this response is an anxious talisman on my part: I know there are people who die of HIV today, even in the developed world, who have done everything they could to be well. It is a terrible thought: one wishes to find some difference from the people who succumb, a sad gesture of denial the human mind almost can't keep itself from making.

I've learned over the years that though I treasure certain possessions there's very little I can't actually live without. I once traveled for many months with just one duffle bag and had such wonderful experiences that I didn't feel I lacked for anything. But of course I can't live without the drugs that play such an enormous role in keeping me alive. I'm deeply grateful for the human ingenuity that developed them and the generosity that makes them available to me and others who couldn't otherwise afford them.

In fact, though there would likely be nothing I could do about it, I do sometimes imagine a time when some national or global crisis would disrupt the pipeline for HIV medications and others. It isn't beyond the range of possibility—a flu epidemic on the scale of 1918, for instance—though in that case, the scale of other tragedies would dwarf a disruption in the supply of my medications. Remember "Y2K," the coding issue that some feared might disrupt computer systems around the world, causing planes to fall out of the sky and banks to collapse? I'm a little embarrassed to remember the conversation I had with my then-pharmacist in Brooklyn about whether he thought I ought to try to stockpile my medications. He looked at me as though I were crazy, and indeed Y2K didn't bring about the Apocalypse, but since then there have in fact been periodic shortages of many kinds of medications, perhaps foreshadowing a more significant disruption in the future.

The network of connections, the social contract, that keeps humanity afloat is not infinitely resilient, as we saw recently when the world economy was driven astonishingly quickly into the ditch. The contract needs to be constantly maintained and reaffirmed in order to continue. Can you tell I'm an aficionado of the worst-case scenario, a worrywart who keeps a hammer in the car for busting out the windows in case I drive off a bridge? This may be a character flaw, but in some ways it has served me well.

The times I spend filling my monthly pillboxes are moments of mystery, awe, and prayer for me: I literally hold in my hand the substances that restrain the virus in my body and that make my life possible. I want these miracle chemicals available for everybody who needs them, and struggle with the question of why I have been selected to receive them. Does anybody remember that years ago actor Malachy McCourt used to answer the phone on his radio call-in show by shouting "YOU HAVE BEEN SELECTED FOR IMMORTALITY"? As I count my pills out, I remember that I've won some strange lottery, just by getting up every morning.

Poetry, good books, music, theater, and art have helped me live my life and given meaning to it. And small human comforts are not by any means irrelevant: when my dental hygienist suggested recently that I give up coffee and tea, I let her know in no uncertain terms that this would not be happening. As poet Jack Gilbert put it, "We can do without pleasure, / but not delight."

A Jewish friend who recovered from cancer and a painful divorce told me once about the prayer called the *Shehecheyanu*: "Blessed are you Lord God, ruler of the universe, who has given us life and sustenance and brought us to this happy season." She said she and her family say this blessing every time they do something for the first time: open the door to a new house, begin a new job, etc. I can't count the times since I contracted HIV that I've felt thankful for having reached this or that day: the day my T-cells first went over 400 (from a nadir of 8), the day I began my graduate study, the day I was awarded my degree, the days my first, second, and third books were accepted for publication. But of all the days, none have been finer than the one in 2002 (my birthday, if you can believe it) on which I met my love, my darling Stephen Miller, and the day in 2005 on which we married in the great Commonwealth of Massachusetts. We both found love late in life, and it's all the more sweet for that. I can't say I feel *proud* to have reached these days, since I played only a small part in that. But I do feel the inexpressible joy that I believe every person takes birth to experience. I hope I have many more years of life and work, but if I were to die tomorrow I could not feel that I have missed anything of life and love, because I have had both in abundance.

There's a certain amount of momentum that one gets from working toward certain professional and personal goals: I have a lot to look forward to, and I think that sends a good message to my immune system. I can't wait till my third book of poems is published, till the second book of Japanese poems Stephen and I have translated together appears, till my poems appear in a well-known journal.

But ego-achievement, nice as it is, can only carry you so far. I get my real strength from the love I give and receive, from the energy the earth and the universe give to all creatures, and from a sense that there is some luminous substance that interpenetrates everything. My life has been hard at times, but I've never felt alone, which I believe is the worst kind of suffering. I've been lucky, lucky, lucky to share my life with superb people, to have experienced much that is beautiful, and to have been led in a path of learning.

Stephen and I had our gold wedding bands inscribed inside with a phrase from William Meredith's poem "Accidents of Birth": "you, to teach me." And we do teach each other, and bring each other back to sanity, every day. As I get older I fall more deeply in love with what I think of as "the human project"—the art, the learning, the achievement, the struggle to become more wise, just, compassionate. Even the weaknesses to which we're susceptible make me feel tenderly about our tribe, and I am so curious about how it all will turn out.

Many of us waste so much time speculating about the future and projecting ourselves into it. Our projections are based on our particular fears and desires, of course, and usually have very little to do with reality. One of the blessings of illness—or, at least, some people are able to turn it into a blessing—is that it can cut short this projection. When we're shown our mortality, we realize that it's impossible to know the future—there are too many variables, most of them beyond our control. We realize that we have only the present, only this moment.

The next question that naturally arises is: "If I have only this moment, what is this moment for?" Everybody has to answer this question for her- or himself, and answering it may be a long and evolving process, if we're lucky enough to be given time for that. But just by causing this question to arise, illness can inspire a powerful reordering of priorities. Things we considered very important, or that we worried a great deal about, may suddenly seem like nothing. Other things that we neglected, or thought we would attend to when we "have the time," may become very important.

Years ago I received a letter from a man who was also recovering from a serious illness. He said that he found himself lethargic, afraid to make plans or begin any new project. Having come so close to death, he wasn't sure how he wanted to spend the rest of his life. A New York psychologist has studied this constellation of symptoms and named it "The Lazarus Syndrome."

I wrote him that I also had had trouble taking up again some of the difficult aspects of my life, which I had felt free of when I thought I was dying. (How to make some money, for instance.) There is a thread that snaps when one lets go of life, and a sense of peaceful relief from struggle. But that thread doesn't break as easily as some people think: I've come to believe it has to be broken, in some sense, with an act of the will. Though sickness may bring us to the brink of death, we have to choose to go. From watching friends die, I came to understand that dying is hard work, just as living is. We have to loosen one by one each of the seals and locks that bind us to the earth plane. As Walt Whitman put it, "Strong is your hold O mortal flesh / Strong is your hold O Love." From my own experience, though I had begun preparing myself to die, I had not yet chosen to, and there was a difference. When I recovered and began to pick up the reins of my life, the fine and difficult both, the life force rose up under me again in all its distressing splendor.

Since then, frustrated as I often get with troubles of my own life or character, there is some part of me that always says *yes* to the speaker of Edna St. Vincent Millay's poem "Renascence":

Ah! Up then from the ground sprang I
And hailed the earth with such a cry
As is not heard save from a man
Who has been dead, and lives again.

I haven't yet touched on why I believe I contracted HIV. The answer is I behaved recklessly in my twenties, but I refuse to condemn the person I was then. I thought little of myself, was fiercely lonely, and turned to regular applications of sexual pleasure to assuage my discomfort. The huge irony isn't lost on me that it took contracting HIV for me to learn how to not throw my life away. I don't struggle against this destiny, because I appreciate the elegant spiritual logic of its design: I had to be shaken awake, and on the whole I'm grateful for the shaking. I would have missed a lot otherwise.

When I was newly diagnosed I was given, or discovered for myself, some advice that proved to be helpful:

Get support: build yourself a "wellness team" that addresses and supports your physical, emotional, and spiritual well-being;

Make whatever changes in your life are necessary to eliminate or lessen threats to your physical, emotional, and spiritual well-being;

Thoroughly educate yourself about HIV and HIV treatment (both conventional and alternative medical approaches) and about general wellness resources like nutrition, vitamin, mineral, and herbal supplements, exercise, and stress management techniques;

Learn what factors help you to be well and assemble as many of those as you can against the stress HIV disease places on your body. Wellness, like disease, is a multifactorial phenomenon; it doesn't arise from one cause. So I've learned to listen to my body, eat well, take supplements, exercise (harder as I get older), manage my stress, address any small problem before it becomes a big one, and to adjust any part of my regimen if it becomes necessary. Part of being a spiritual warrior in reference to any disease means arming yourself with knowledge and not expecting your medical providers to have all the answers. This is even more important for people who don't live in urban areas where doctors are familiar with HIV standard-of-care: frequently since I left New York I find myself asking for tests or treatments that are not common in the areas where I now live. I'm not shy about advocating for myself in such situations.

Some medical professionals give lip service to the idea that they're happy to work with well-informed patients who expect to play an important role in making decisions about their own health care. In fact and in practice, such doctors are less common than I wish: not too many years ago I was even "fired" by one doctor because I was and am assertive in asking questions, weighing alternatives, and choosing treatment plans that make sense for me and my life. I, in turn, have left (or not joined) medical practices that were not up to date with what I understand as standard-of-care. I interview doctors at first appointments as an educated consumer. If that surprises or angers some individual doctors, so be it: if I don't get a good feeling, or receive answers that I feel aren't optimal, I move on. One doctor, at our first meeting, replied to a question with the answer "If I answer that question, you'll just have more questions." I never went back there, and if necessary I travel to access the best care rather than settle for less.

Some patients encourage paternalistic behavior on the part of doctors by giving them an almost godlike power and authority and by not taking responsibility for those parts of their own lives that are in their control. To such patients I say, educate yourself, keep good records, go to every appointment prepared to ask questions, to learn, and to weigh alternatives. To such doctors I say, become willing to work with feisty and knowledgeable patients.

Over the last three decades men and women with HIV and women with breast cancer, among others, have virtually forced some autocratic doctors, hospitals, and drug companies to improve the way they relate to patients, at least in the United States. We've forced them to see us as people rather than as cogs in the vast health-care enterprise. But we still have a long way to go until people with life-challenging illness receive the care they need in the context of fully respectful and *human* relationships with medical professionals.

We who are living with life-challenging illness have an important role to play in this, not only by educating and standing up for ourselves, but by becoming activist about helping others receive the treatments they need. Many is the time that I fought for some test or treatment—and got it—and afterward thought: what if I had not known what to fight for, or how to fight, as must be the case with many? Many patients walk away after having been told *no*, not realizing that pressing harder might have meant a different answer. Insurance companies, Medicare, Medicaid, Social Security, and private disability institutions, in particular, count on our meekness and lack of information: it saves them money and effort. My advice is, don't make it easier for them. Get smart for yourself, then share what you know with people in a similar situation. There is almost always a way over, around, or underneath any given obstacle, given enough stubbornness.

Though in my years navigating the health care system I've been frustrated with a small number of individual doctors, there are many stellar doctors and organizations who are leading the way toward a more holistic view of medical care and the relationship between doctor and patient, and also to the integration of medicine with access to food, shelter, clean water, sanitation, education, and economic opportunities.

One is Paul Farmer, who by founding Partners in Health has changed the way HIV, TB and other formerly fatal diseases are treated around the world today. I give to them every chance I get.

I keep a framed quote on a shelf in the meditation room that Stephen and I have set up in our house. It's from an essay by James Carse and expresses perfectly what I've come to feel about living with HIV, or about any other danger that threatens to diminish my life:

> This is the deepest secret of the living water: it transforms every obstruction into a new expression of itself. It accepts as channel what is presented as barrier. The mountain does not stand in the way of the spring; it is the way of the spring.

# Type One

RILEY PASSMORE

I was sixteen when I told my mother I didn't want to die.

I don't remember much of that time, those two weeks when my body was eating itself alive, desperate for insulin, desperate, ironically, for simple sugars and complex carbohydrates, but I remember that. I remember her face. She tried not to flinch when I said what I said. She tried not to let her terror show. But I know my mother, and I know that when she purses her lips into a thin red line and looks away, as though to find a distraction, she is afraid.

She hugged me tight, using the embrace to hide her expression.

"It's like nothing sticks," I said, referring to food and drink. I had been urinating fully every half-hour for the last three days, and I had not eaten in a week. Despite my untreated diabetes reducing my body mass to a skeletal 108 pounds, I was not hungry. The sugar trapped in my blood told my body I was full, and my body, stupid as it was, believed it, choosing instead to dump the excess sugar into my kidneys and out, uselessly, through my toilet.

Little did I know, though, that she already knew what was wrong, my mother, that the lab technician handling my bloodwork had already called my primary care physician, who had already called the pediatric endocrinologist, who then had already called my mother.

The rationale was to spare my feelings, I later heard.

The doctors, the nurses, my mother—they did not want to frighten me.

I used to think their sentiment was so silly, that they should have just told me then and there, over the phone, while I was at home, sleeping twenty hours a day, my mother and my father and my brother at work and at school. I probably wouldn't have understood the person on the other end anyway, as delirious as I was. For all I knew, the flu was to blame.

But when my mother drove home early from work to take me to the emergency room, having to carry me out like an infant to her still-running sedan, I could see why. As she closed the passenger-side door I finally caught a glimpse of my face in the rear-view, the face of an emaciated teenager who hadn't shaved in weeks, his hair thick and bushy and wild. He was utterly unrecognizable, even though he was me, with sunken cheeks and yellow skin, with week-old pajamas hanging off his wasting frame like the bed sheets of a Halloween ghost. No parent of any strength would ever want to name an episode like that for her son. No parent would ever want to say its name aloud, the name of the Devil who was killing their child.

For when we name something, when we give something—even suffering, especially suffering—a title, a designation, a nomenclature, we make that something real. We create it, forge it, with nothing more than the flutter of our lips and the exhalation of our breath. And then, like magic, that something, that suffering, becomes permanent. Immutable.

Like a diagnosis, never to be changed again.

# The Bad Patient

SANDRA BEASLEY

Because after chatting about his child's food allergies for ten min-utes, that distinctive ache has stirred at the back of my throat, yet I say nothing. The restaurant manager has been kind. He prides himself on taking care of customers like me. Because a reaction often begins with swallowing—repeated, reflexive—I drain a glass of water and finish my wine. Vegan cuisine conveniently avoids dairy or egg, beef, and shrimp, but steers me smack into the path of cucumbers, mango, tofu, tree nuts. The sauce I thought was tahini might be cashew butter. I put the wrap down and take a Benadryl. I take another Benadryl a minute later.

I leave most of the second sauvignon blanc on the table and tip big.

I walk out alone. I arrived alone. It is a Sunday night in South Beach and I don't live in South Beach, or Miami, or even Florida. I have a full twenty-block walk ahead, but if I don't move my car before getting help it'll be towed tomorrow morning.

I get behind the wheel. As I turn from the quiet of Washington Avenue to the buzz of Collins, I realize I cannot drive. The friend I call on my cell phone can't make out my words as I describe my location. I yank myself out of the right lane and into a fancy hotel's driveway, open the door, and vomit onto the pavement. When I look at the startled valet, the first thing I say is: "I'm not drunk."

*Where is your EpiPen?* I have had the epinephrine injector with me the whole time—at the restaurant, on my walk, in the car, at the hotel, and in my friends' car as they drive me to the hospital. I have carried an EpiPen in my purse, carrying that purse room to room wherever I go, for almost thirty years. I just don't opt to use it. Again.

Sheldon Kaplan, a biomedical engineer who also designed a medical kit for the Apollo Moon Missions, invented the EpiPen. A spring-loaded needle releases epinephrine directly into muscle, ideally the fleshy thigh, where it acts more quickly than if ingested by pill or patch. The first crystalline "epinephrine," created in 1897, was extracted from a sheep's adrenal glands. Today's version is entirely synthetic. Although the benefits of adrenaline had been observed for decades, including an ability to increase blood pressure and relax the muscles lining airways, it wasn't until the 1960s that scientists identified receptor molecules that trigger these cellular responses. This research earned Robert J. Lefkowitz and Brian K. Kobilka the 2012 Nobel Prize in Chemistry.

The EpiPen went on the commercial market in 1980, the year I was born. It was prescribed for treating anaphylactic reactions, a phenomenon that was considered rare at the time, defined primarily in terms of cardiac distress and difficulty breathing. If you carried an EpiPen because you were allergic to bee stings or penicillin, anaphylaxis was an imminent threat; you knew to inject yourself the moment you swatted at your skin and came away with a stinger in your hand.

If, like me, you carried an EpiPen as a bulwark against multiple food allergies—some severe, some mild, some still unknown—the guidelines were murkier. Every bite into a new fruit or vegetable is a test of my system. Every bite into a prepackaged snack or restaurant dish carries the risk of cross-contamination. A food that does not trigger a reaction the first time I eat it might trigger a reaction the second time, or the ninth.

During childhood reactions, thirty years ago, my lips would hive up, or my eyelids would swell. I might make a *squonk-ee* noise that my parents recognized as an effort to scratch my itching throat. I might feel "bubbles" of irritation along my esophagus or queasiness in my stomach. I might feel feverish. If I'd eaten enough of the offending food I could throw up, though usually I'd only had a single bite or two. Occasionally the reaction began before I'd even swallowed.

Despite all these things, if I was coherent and alert, answering questions and neither hypoxic nor incontinent, we rode it out. I took antihistamines, usually Benadryl. Sometimes my grandfather or uncle, both naval doctors, would come by the house to check on me. I'd feel the cool moon of a stethoscope pressed against my breastbone.

Other times we decided to go to the hospital. The nursing staff did a lot of watching; we did a lot of waiting. Even after a first reaction recedes, many hospitals will hold you in case there is a second, biphasic reaction four to eight hours later. Epinephrine was a possibility, but more often I was administered a corticosteroid to suppress my immune system—the first of what would be several days' worth of prednisone. The dosing of prednisone has improved since the eighties and nineties. Back then it was PMS in a pill, an instant gain of five pounds water and ten pounds bitchiness.

Often, if I tell stories of these reactions to parents, they ask, "And when did you use your EpiPen?" I pause, knowing I am about to disappoint them, and look across the divide of a generation. For them epinephrine is first response. For us it was last resort.

I meet these parents in bookstores, in schools, at literary festivals. We find each other because I've written a memoir that doubles as a cultural history of food allergy. "A memoir," I remind them, "not a manual."

Before the book, I had not spent much time with the advocacy communities around allergy. There were once two that dominated the American conversation—the Food Allergy & Anaphylaxis Network, founded in 1991 and based in Virginia, and the Food Allergy

Initiative, founded in 1998 and headquartered in New York. Though their missions looked similar in the abstract, they differed substantively in tone. FAAN was family-oriented, providing resources and guides for everyday life; FAI focused on policy and research. In 2012 they fused to become FARE: Food Allergy Research & Education.

In December 2011 I was invited to attend the Food Allergy Initiative's ball in New York City. I hadn't been to a black-tie event in years. I grabbed a column dress hanging at the back of my closet that I'd first used for a dance as a high school freshman, wadded the velvet into an overnight bag, and rode the Amtrak train up from D.C.

I would have been disappointed if I'd arrived at the gala expecting to eat, but I would've also been naïve. I stopped for sushi on my way to the Waldorf Astoria. In the Grand Ballroom canopied with tiny lights, I demurred when offered dry-aged steak with "marrow mustard custard" and onion rings in a French wine sauce. I nervously adjusted the straps of my dress and made small talk. I was seated across from a renowned allergist; to be precise, I was seated across from his teenage son. Audra McDonald and Norm Lewis came out to sing selections from *The Gershwins' Porgy and Bess*.

Later I read that the five hundred guests in attendance raised $4.5 million for "the cause of food allergies." What is the "cause" of food allergies? Many in the room were focused on supporting studies of OIT, oral immunotherapy, and SLIT, sublingual immunotherapy. These treatments aim to desensitize patients through graduated exposure to an allergen. A successful trial outcome might be a peanut-allergic child who, after ingesting small doses of peanut flour daily, with slight increases every two weeks for months, achieves a sustained tolerance of four grams: a dozen peanuts, give or take.

OIT and SLIT are experimental and time-consuming and their outcomes, for now, are largely academic. We don't know how we would adapt these procedures for those with multiple food allergies, or those at increased risk of anaphylaxis from even the slightest exposure. The cynic in me thinks of Whac-a-Mole—three years of my life spent acclimating to cashews, great. Now what about pistachios? Milk? Shrimp?

But for those most likely to donate to food allergy research, immunotherapy offers a crucial commodity: the promise of a cure. I sat in the Waldorf Astoria surrounded by smart, wealthy, dedicated people who wanted very badly to fix their children. Which made me feel, in a way I had not before, just a little bit broken.

I put my overnight bag over one arm and, over the other arm, slung the FAI tote with the leather handles and embossed insignia. Inside were pamphlets, a houndstooth-print umbrella, and snacks with exceptionally clear ingredient labeling. Later that night I would stand tippy-toe, arms outstretched, and rotate to show off my dress to a friend. He wolf-whistled for effect. On the walk to his studio he pointed out an oversized plastic Santa Claus face, glowing from a brownstone's lower level. In the photo, arching myself to the curve of Santa's jolly, bulb-lit beard, you can't even tell I'm clothed. We lay in his bed. We talked about his girlfriend. I moved to the couch. The next morning, walking to the subway, I tried to avoid catching the heels of my silver stilettos in the sidewalk grates.

In 1973 Pentagon officials approached Survival Technologies, Inc., Sheldon Kaplan's employer. They needed a new kind of injection device. The stainless-steel chamber used in existing injection designs was not a stable combination with certain nerve agent antidotes. Kaplan got to work. Four years later his team filed patent 4,031,893 for "Hypodermic injection device having means for varying the medicament capacity thereof." STI delivered the ComboPen to the Department of Defense. They began to ready the EpiPen for consumer sale.

During the seventies someone with severe allergies might have carried an Ana-Kit, introduced to the market by Hollister-Stier. The kit's preloaded ampoules eliminated the guesswork of drawing epinephrine into a syringe in the middle of an allergic reaction; however, they did little to alleviate the anxiety of handling a needle. Kaplan's injector both hides the needle, a larger gauge to punch through clothing, and amplifies the force with which it thrusts into the body. The toughest part might be steadying an EpiPen for the three-full-Mississippi seconds it takes to deploy its contents. You can't just swing and jab; people who jerk away have ended up with lacerations, the thick needle slicing through the skin. I'm sure it hurts. Dying would hurt more.

In 1986 the average wholesale cost of an EpiPen was about $36. By the late 1990s, when I remember accompanying my mother to the pharmacy to refill our annual prescription, we paid $50. This was a significant expense but not an insurmountable one. Then in 2007 the EpiPen product was acquired by the Mylan corporation as part of an aggressive global expansion that included purchasing Merck KGaA's entire generics business, as well as a controlling interest in Matrix Laboratories, which supplied active pharmaceutical ingredients. In the subsequent decade Mylan turned the sale of EpiPens from a $2-million-dollar-per-year business into more than a billion dollars of annual revenue. Their product has the built-in obsolescence of a one-year shelf life, which is fruitful, but that has long been the case. How did Mylan create a 29% compound annual growth rate in sales?

The surge in EpiPen purchases was, in part, a reflection of allergy's growing prevalence in the population. A 2007 Centers for Disease Control and Prevention survey identified 4% of Americans under age eighteen as having food allergies; then a 2011 study, published in the journal *Pediatrics*, put the figure at 8%, or one out of thirteen kids. Most states, particularly after several rounds of lobbying at the congressional level, now require that school clinics stock epinephrine injectors. Many private businesses, such as theme parks and cruise ships, have added them to their in-house dispensary. I like to know EpiPens are nestled in first-aid kits, just as I like to see automated external defibrillators on the walls at airports. But increased demand is just part of the picture.

In 2011, citing federal guidelines that advised carrying two epinephrine dosages at all times, based on case studies where patients continued to react after the first injection, Mylan discontinued the option of buying single injectors. Your kid misplaces one while at his soccer game? You can only afford one on this paycheck, but plan to buy another next month? Tough. Get two at a time, or none at all.

Fair market competition has often been lacking. While other pharmaceutical companies have offered EpiPen clones, they haven't been successful. Auvi-Q was recalled; the Food and Drug Administration cited a generic model proposed by Teva Pharmaceuticals as having "major deficiencies." Twinject was discontinued; eventually this evolved to become Adrenaclick. The Amedra Pharmaceuticals' product has potential but little market muscle. Sooner or later something will break through—or maybe consumers will simply flock to the generic model promised by Mylan. In the meantime, EpiPen has had 85% of the epinephrine injector market using a prohibitive price point.

When I came up to the register at the Kaiser Permanente on Capitol Hill to pick up my prescription in early 2016, the pharmacist shook her head and exhaled. "Did you know what this was going to cost?" she asked. $381.23. More than my paycheck. I paused for a minute, a minute that would have been punctuated by my mother's howl had she been there to see me balk. Then I pulled out the credit card I'd been trying to pay off.

When I mentioned sticker shock to others later, people I didn't even realize had allergies spoke up. One friend had been given an estimated price of $600 after insurance, $800 before. One of my students admitted she has never been able to afford an EpiPen. She always tries to be within fifteen minutes of a hospital.

As with any medical condition, the individual narrative is shaped by class economics. Even if you've got a working EpiPen in hand, using it means a four- to twenty-four-hour hospital stay, which could equal a childcare crisis or losing a job. Recent studies in the United States, the United Kingdom, and Australia all show rising admissions for allergic reactions, with the highest incidence rate corresponding to younger patients. Perhaps that's because of sheer volume; more children are allergic than ever before. Yet I wonder if twenty years from now, when those children have become adults in their own right, we will still see a leveling off of admissions in older patients. The truth is that the decisions our parents make for us are not the same decisions we make for ourselves.

A few years ago I traveled to Georgia for the AJC-Decatur Book Festival. I met a friend before my afternoon panel—a reading from the food allergy memoir—and we sat down for lunch at a farm-to-table restaurant that was a favorite of the participating authors. The roasted chicken with fingerling potatoes was delicious. Was it a touch too greasy-good? Only at the very end, as I sopped up the *jus*, did my lips begin to tingle. A faint rushing noise dialed up, a buzzing. I looked around to see if anyone else could hear it. My gut surged. I slipped a Benadryl into my palm, then my mouth. I kept talking to my friend and my friend's friend, who was telling the story of a nasty divorce.

If I bailed on the panel, I would be violating my festival contract. Would they ask me to pay for the hotel room? There was no opportunity to delay, no do-overs.

I called the waitress over and, in the guise of praising the dish, asked her to describe the exact details of preparation. As she listed herbs and spices, stocks and vinegars and oils, nothing about the story had changed. The kitchen knew about my allergies. That meant the culprit was probably accidental, a dirty spoon or spatula. I swallowed hard, excused myself to the bathroom to scrub my lips with a wad of toilet paper, and went to my panel. When the next day's lunch date asked about a location, I said, "I know a really good place." To change it up, I tried the trout and couscous.

When caretakers dominate the advocacy conversation, disconnects are inevitable. Sometimes this is a matter of demanding a service without fully anticipating the consequences: a parent insists on a "peanut-free" table for her child but does not ask her child if anyone else is allergic. The child sits alone during every lunch for a year. Sometimes this is a matter of not anticipating the need for a service at all.

One major blind spot in the food-allergic advocacy community is alcohol. If a body is primed to react to an ingredient, the body does not care whether that ingredient is delivered via a fork or a martini glass. Olives comes stuffed with everything from almonds to bleu cheese to anchovies, which are three of America's "Big Eight" allergen categories. Labels on liqueurs and craft beers do not always clarify the source of their flavorings, nor are they required to, because the Food and Drug Administration does not oversee alcoholic products. Sangrias are topped off with cubes of mango and melon; pisco sours are foamed with egg white; garnish cutting boards and cocktail shakers are reused without anything more than a quick rinse.

The irony is that these dangers might be occurring at the very restaurants that pride themselves on being sensitive to food allergies. Often a drink order is taken the moment the customer sits down—before he or she has even thought to share any dietary restrictions or request a "nut-free" menu. In 2012 the National Restaurant Association released SERVSafe Allergens, an interactive online training course designed to ensure that restaurants have informed and sensitive staff. But nowhere in the program is bar prep a source of concern. All the attention is on front and back of the house, the waiters and the kitchen crew. The National Restaurant Association consulted with FARE while creating the SERVSafe program; how did no one flag this as an issue? But FARE, whose offices are dominated by concerned parents, tends to focus on threats posed to those under the legal drinking age.

When I wrote about this for a newspaper, a category of commenter threaded their sympathy with disdain. C'mon, they suggested, these are not inalienable rights. Skip the booze for a night.

I've never been afraid of needles, but I am conscious of the bruises they cause, to the point of vetoing intravenous fluids. Phlebotomists have told me I'm a tough draw and that I should always request a "butterfly," a winged infusion set. Once, after a routine test, I came home and took a long bath. I held the punctured crook of my arm under the flow of hot water, not realizing the pressure I was putting on the fresh clot, and screamed when I saw blood flare wide under the surface of the skin.

For a hemophiliac there is no such thing as a routine bruise or bleed. In *Codeine Diary: True Confessions of a Reckless Hemophiliac,* author Tom Andrews reflects on the tension between being a writer who happens to have a disease versus being a diseased individual who happens to write. He recognizes the peril of setting himself up as a professional hemophiliac, "recklessly confident that I speak for all bleeders."

He opens his memoir with a fall on the ice. What he should do is head straight to the hospital, cooling the injury along the way, to receive an infusion of factor VIII or desmopressin as soon as possible. What he does, instead, is take the bus back to his apartment. He frames the unfolding narrative in these terms:

> I have not chosen an "ideal" bleed. That is, there is much about my reaction to the traumatized ankle and about my interaction with doctors that I am not proud of. "Warts and all or not at all" was my guiding principle. There is occasional pettiness, and childishness, on my part. There is spinelessness. There is misguided anger. Above all, there is the flurry of thought and fear, which eventually gives way to the surprising, implausible surge of convalescence, the spirit's if not the body's, a convergence of self and world that opens one's eyes to the mysterious in the familiar after a season in hell.

The "season in hell" is a hospital-bedded, codeine-mitigated haze during which he lavishes appreciation on his wife, riffs on John Ashbery and Joe Brainard, recalls setting a world record, and confronts memories of his brother's death from kidney disease.

Andrews's stream-of-consciousness during his initial emergency treatment disturbs me because its extremes are so familiar. First come what he calls the "reality orientation" exercises: the rehearsal of who you are, how old you are, where you are, who you're with, why you're there, and other willfully banal observations. I always do this aloud, as tangible confirmation that my airway is open. Then comes what he calls the "ontological breakdown," the moment in which selfhood begins to slip. You become a metaphor, a construct. Your pain is a bow, sliding slowly across the neck of a violin. Though, unlike Andrews, I've never then bargained for Darvon or morphine. Anaphylaxis frightens, but it doesn't burn and pulse the way a fractured, bleeding joint does.

The final section of his memoir, "On Being a Bad Insurance Risk," interrogates the social contract thrust upon those with chronic illness. We heed. We obey. We comply with treatments based on what may be still-evolving science. Andrews receives transfusions on the front end of medicine's comprehension of HIV as a blood-borne disease. He ultimately tests negative, but his anxiety is palpable. "I can well imagine God's spitting at my prayer of thanks for being passed over by AIDS," he writes.

We are expected to be the best versions of ourselves. We are at the mercy of minor chance events. "Once, I lifted a gallon of milk in such a way as to break a blood vessel in my elbow," Andrews writes. "The joint's interior filled with blood until my elbow looked like a steroid-enhanced eggplant." Once I sat down with my parents at an Italian bar and we were offered a dish of olives. Who looks at a dish of olives and asks, "Are you sure these aren't buttered?"

Andrews originally imagines his book closing with thoughts of John, his dead brother, and the notion of sea changes, "the impor-

tance of 'being well while ill.'" Instead the book plunges ahead
with the confession that Andrews, divorced, has recently bought
a Kawasaki KLX 250 bike. In his inaugural competition he crashes
four times. This comes twenty years after overshooting a corner
in a motocross race, suffering a punctured calf muscle from the
bike's foot peg, and being begged by his parents and hematologist
to stop. "I was about to race motocross again," he writes, "because
I needed to affirm that I was still an amateur hemophiliac, that I
hadn't turned pro."

Is that what I'm trying to be? A resolute amateur?

"Our culture urges people with chronic illnesses to resolve rich
tensions," he writes, "that to my mind are better left unresolved."

Solutions of epinephrine are not supposed to be left in tempera-
tures lower than 59 degrees or higher than 86 degrees. For some
that simply means protecting them while at the beach, or skiing,
or other isolated occurrences. For others the daily conditions of
work—harvesting a field of corn or pouring concrete at an outdoor
construction site—render the auto-injector an impractical accessory
even while it remains a critical one.

I think of this because my husband, an artist, sometimes works an
hourly-wage job building rain gardens. We make sure his lunches
are vegetarian because meat can spoil during the morning's work.
The first few times he mentioned calling in sick because the tem-
peratures were predicted to top 95 degrees, he took my silence as
judgment. Not judgment so much as frustration, I told him. Two
years into our joint insurance plan he still had not seen a doctor,
meaning the $300 a month we pay on his behalf had gone entirely
unutilized. He needed a physical. He needed a baseline measure of
his health. He's a man in his upper forties, and of course he should
be careful of manual labor on a scorching day. My hypocrisy, as I
said all this, was bitter in the mouth.

At age eleven Tom Andrews got into the *Guinness Book of World
Records* by clapping his hands 94,520 times for fourteen hours

and thirty-one minutes straight. He raced motocross; he practiced stand-up routines; he was diagnosed with hemophilia; he wrote *Codeine Diary;* he rode a bike again. He died in 2001, at age forty, after a coma related to contracting thrombotic thrombocytopenic purpura, a rare coagulation disorder. He had no health insurance at the time.

As an undergraduate at the University of Virginia I read Andrews's collection, *The Hemophiliac's Motorcycle.* The experience was a kind of paradigm shift, as I began to consider how chronic illness could shape an author's voice rather than being a footnote. Not that I was ready to be shaped myself. It would be a few years until I'd wrangle with the medicalized body on the page in a sequence called "Allergy Girl."

A few of us from undergrad workshops stayed in touch. Morgan and I traded emails, each slightly embarrassed to have never known about the other's illness while at UVA: my allergies, his cystic fibrosis. Perhaps I should have guessed from his drafts, as if images of snow settling over branches are actually secretions blanketing the bronchi and alveoli. Or not. He had moved to Arizona, where he got an MFA degree, taught, ran a small press, and published chapbooks, including one titled $L=u=N=G=U=A=G=E$.

The cruelty of cystic fibrosis is that when a lung transplant becomes necessary—which it usually does, as function declines—both lungs must go. Otherwise, lingering bacteria can infect a fresh, healthy organ. Morgan went into surgery at the end of 2011. On January 30, 2012, he passed away at age thirty-three.

"I almost die a lot," I said last year, for some forgettable reason, a quick quip for a laugh. For nights after, I sat with those words. I've weathered dozens of reactions over the years, which makes calling my condition "life-threatening" seem like indulgence. Few things annoy me more than when a well-meaning dinner companion interjects with an announcement to emphasize the seriousness of my requests: "She could die, you know."

Yet the prescriptive attitude toward anaphylaxis is that any allergic episode can be the one that kills you. The formula for acceptable response is rigid: you shoot the epinephrine. You go straight to the hospital. If you're not amenable to those terms, it can be hard to know how to enter the societal conversation.

*Now, I have learned to be a bad patient,* I wrote in a poem.

A few years back I met my dad for a happy hour on M Street in northwest Washington. He had fed the meter for two hours without a destination in mind, and we descended the steps to Vidalia. The southern-themed restaurant was deserted this early in the evening and workweek. We ordered drinks and began to navigate the menu with the bartender, only to be interrupted by a curt, volcanic man wearing whites. He slapped a dishrag down on the counter. "What are you allergic to?" he asked.

I only got to mention the foods I always mention first—milk, egg—before he said, "You good with pig?" We nodded and he disappeared. Twenty minutes later he walked out with a terrine of pork. There were cornichons and mustard seeds on the cutting board's side; I could eat around those. But what assurance did I have that there wasn't another random ingredient? Shrimp, or beef? The man stared at us expectantly.

"Thank you," I said, and took a tiny bite. Then, after a few minutes, another bite.

I had never eaten anything like that before, nor have I since. He didn't know the extraordinary extent of my allergies. I didn't know that he had received a James Beard award in the category of Best Chef Mid-Atlantic. I did not have a reaction. Luck. Terrines, I have since learned, frequently contain pistachios. There is no moral to this story.

I am not a bad patient. I am not a good patient. I'm a person who is weighing the risk of dying against the needs of living, day by day. I'm not the only one.

# A Tribute to the Pharmacist

TAISON BELL

Dear Pharmacist,

You just paged me and, I must admit, I'm not feeling excited to call back. I estimate that I probably get paged, called, texted, or stopped in person by you exactly $X \cdot 10^2$ per day, where "X" is the number of days I've been on service. Despite all of the interactions over the years, I have never stopped to really consider our relationship. Here are a few of our most memorable moments:

You once paged me while I was driving home from clinic. I had just finished a hellish day filled with overbooked patients, prior authorization requests, and last-minute walk-ins. I was relieved just to make it to the end without pulling my hair out (and I'm bald). I finished seeing my last patient, whom I diagnosed with pneumonia and prescribed a fluoroquinolone. You called to ask me if I wanted to change the patient's multivitamin from the morning to the evening, since ("as you know") taking supplements that include divalent cations with fluoroquinolones render the antibiotic ineffective. "Of course!" I said, "Thank you for 'reminding' me." Meanwhile I took a moment to file that away, because—as a so-called infectious disease specialist—that's probably something I should already know. I've learned many helpful tips like this from you over the years.

You once paged me while I was working in the ICU. I was admitting a patient to the unit in wide-open septic shock and multi-organ failure. In fact I had just finished intubating, placing two central lines, placing an arterial line, and writing dialysis orders—all in just 1.5 hours! I was fist-bumping the nurses and feeling on top of the world; and, just as my head was expanding with the rare moment to stroke my ego, I received your page. You reminded me that, despite being the day's Procedure King/Line-master, this awesomeness didn't prevent me from ordering the wrong diluent for the vasopressin. You asked if I could "kindly" reorder it so that the patient could—you know, while I'm celebrating—actually have a blood pressure that was compatible with life? During our history you've been able to refocus my energy and avert errors multiple times.

You were once rounding with me and my team. You politely demurred when I incorrectly stated that (*insert gobbledygook*)-umab was a new monoclonal antibody that inhibits the RAOP (random and obscure protein) pathway to do something I don't quite understand but am told is good for MGUS. You waited until I had finished stumbling through my rather weak teaching point to correct the record. By the end I could only muster, "At least I got the monoclonal antibody part right." Though I remember busting my tail in medical school pharmacology, it seems that most of what I learned is now either outdated or irrelevant (I'm still waiting for the day I get to use methyldopa in a pregnant patient). To be honest, I can't keep up with the new drugs as well as I would like to—especially the monoclonal antibodies, which seem to be multiplying like mogwais caught in a rainstorm. Since I began my training, you've helped keep me up to date when I fall behind.

To all of my pharmacy colleagues: It's important for me to acknowledge the critical role you play in the care of my patients. Integrating pharmacists into patient care teams leads to better patient outcomes for diabetes, congestive heart failure, urgent care and hospitalization, inpatient length of stay, and a host of other conditions and metrics. Many of these studies also show that the benefits come while decreasing healthcare costs. Despite clear evidence that they contribute to improved outcomes, a survey of pharmacists shows that a majority report job-related stress due to role ambiguity and conflict with providers. After speaking to several pharmacists I learned that they are often left feeling like an annoyance to doctors and nurses as a result of their interactions with us. So despite knowing how important their job is, many feel underappreciated.

So while the pharmacists are rounding on their special rolling tables labeled "For Pharmacist Only," their laptops loaded with software I've never seen, heads down and toiling away, it's important to recognize that they directly contribute to saving lives, improving outcomes, and making it all more affordable. It is far better for us, and most importantly for our patients, to have them around making up for our shortcomings and pushing us to deliver the highest quality patient care.

So I will make a promise: the next time I hear "Pharmacy on line 3," instead of using my rehearsed "What is it *now*" voice delivered with a perfectly flat affect, I'll listen courteously, assure you that I will check a QTC before giving that dose of Haldol, and thank you for the good work that you do.

Sincerely,
Your Colleague

# Flying into Jerusalem

KATHERINE MACFARLANE

Sometimes, when I'm absentmindedly thinking of how many months are left in the school year, what might have been hits me hard. I was supposed to be pregnant by now.

The first time someone asked me when I was going to have a baby, I was on my honeymoon. Three and a half years later the interest in my womb persists. We still don't have kids. There are lots of reasons why we've waited.

I wasn't ready.

It was the wrong time.

I felt like I'd just left childhood behind myself.

The questions about "when" really bugged me. I had to get some indignation out of my system. So I started writing on my Facebook wall in the voice of a character I called "the Empty Uterus."

After Thanksgiving the Empty Uterus posted: "Nope, just ate a really big piece of turkey and am still loading up on leftovers. Bloated, but not pregnant."

The Empty Uterus feigned surprise when presented with common knowledge: "You're kidding. It's harder to have kids after you turn 35? But my 35th birthday is less than 9 months away!"

"Still empty," was my favorite Empty Uterus aside.

Is involuntary childlessness funny? Everyone seemed to think so. But beneath all this joking, a plan was underway to get a baby into that empty uterus.

But because I have rheumatoid arthritis ("RA"), like all of my major life choices, this plan had multiple steps and contingency plans. First, I had to test run how my body would react to going off some of the medication I was taking labeled "Category X," which is not safe for a fetus.

One such medication is methotrexate. I'd been on it for about twenty years—since I was a preteen. Not only is methotrexate Category X, but at high dosages it's used to induce abortion. If you get pregnant while on methotrexate, the pregnancy might be ectopic, or, if a baby can be delivered, serious birth defects result. What most rheumatologists tell women my age about methotrexate is that "you can't get pregnant on methotrexate!" but the real advice should be "you must use birth control on methotrexate!"

You can't just stop taking methotrexate. That poison lingers.

"Six months is safest to make sure methotrexate is out of your system," one doctor told me.

"Three months is fine!" said doctor two.

I chose the six-month approach. January, the month of resolutions, was my first methotrexate-free month. At first I felt no different. Then, around February, I flared. I struggled to walk and had to use a cane for a few weeks. But otherwise the methotrexate elimination went well. I didn't miss it.

At the same time I was going off methotrexate, I was getting pressured to stop taking Plaquenil, a powerful medicine known as a "disease modifier." My ophthalmologist was concerned that I'd taken it for so long that the accumulation of Plaquenil in my system could trigger Plaquenil-induced blindness. Because I have iritis, glaucoma, and macular edema issues in addition to RA, there's no good reason to risk making my eyes worse.

My rheumatologist resisted, wanting to keep me on Plaquenil, so the compromise was to halve my dosage. The rheumatologist never actually talked to the ophthalmologist. I negotiated the happy medium myself.

The weather got warmer and I started spending more time out-doors. I can't walk that far, but I can swim for miles. I'd hit up an outdoor pool for a few hours, and as I toweled off noticed strange brown splotches on my forehead and nose, as though my skin was tanning but only in random spots.

"I have a skin fungus!" I told my husband.

"You have a sunburn," he said.

The one thing I've had going for me since adolescence is relatively good skin. All of a sudden I looked like I'd faked-and-baked too long at a Myrtle Beach strip mall.

"This is what we call 'The Mask of Pregnancy,'" the dermatologist told me.

"WHAT?"

"No, you're not pregnant," the doctor said, chuckling. Because being or not being pregnant is just so hilarious.

"What you have is similar to the skin markings we see on women who are pregnant. Yours is from Plaquenil. It's making you pho-tosensitive."

So no more Plaquenil.

By June, six months into my getting-ready-to-try phase, I was off Plaquenil and methotrexate, but still on Remicade, a chemothera-peutic agent infused every eight weeks through an IV, in addition to the potent steroid prednisone. I was swimming and writing. The pain was manageable. I was feeling good for once. "I can do this," I thought.

Then I crashed. The pain of a sudden, intense flare woke me up at night. My joints throbbed and I couldn't straighten out my arms or my legs. My joints were locked.

On top of the usual (swollen knees, perma-bent left elbow), my hips were aching. I couldn't climb stairs—I was pulling myself up them. I'd get stuck on the toilet, unable to use my legs or my weakened arms to pull myself up. Pain like this is exhausting. I was dragging myself through my days.

I went on a Medrol pack, which pumps high doses of steroids into my system, and it worked for about a week. The day after the pills ran out, my knees swelled again. I packed on about ten pounds, which meant that once school started in August most of my clothes didn't fit.

This was my pregnancy dry run. It was a disaster.

All of this came as something of a surprise. Ever since I brought up the subject of motherhood fifteen years ago, my doctors had given me vague assurances that pregnancy would never be a problem. That RA would not rob me of this experience. Year after year no doctor could think of any reason why I shouldn't or couldn't conceive. They encouraged me to do so sooner rather than later, before I hit thirty-five—the same advice my friends were getting.

But I was in a downward spiral and I wasn't even pregnant yet. No one had told me about this part.

The thing is, conception is one thing, and that's all my doctors were focused on. Maybe that's what they thought I cared about. But pregnancy, for me, is about much more than fertility. It may mean losing my ability to walk due to medication changes—I might flare before, during, and, if I choose to breastfeed and continue to stay off certain medications, after, a baby's arrival.

Independent of the medication changes, I could have pregnancy-induced flares.

"You'll go into remission," one doctor told me, painting an idyllic picture of what pregnancy would be like.

Some women with autoimmune diseases do experience a lessening of symptoms during pregnancy. Most autoimmune disease drugs are designed to suppress the patient's autoimmune system. Pregnancy itself suppresses the body's natural immune response to a baby's presence, so the experience of being pregnant may, as a side effect, mimic the drugs I take for RA.

But the chances of that happening are, at best, one in three. And even if I experienced that nine-month reprieve, it still wouldn't resolve the pre- and post-pregnancy medication changes I'd have to make.

Still, all of this information wasn't going to stop me! The doctors said I could do it! On I went.

*Half a league, half a league,*
*Half a league onward.*

In July I asked my doctor to order a bone density scan to see how much worse my hips had gotten in the past eighteen months. It revealed that my right hip was now in the throes of osteoporosis, and that my left hip was on its way to the same fate.

I've been on prednisone for twenty-four years, so in some ways, this is no surprise, but it's never easy to hear that you have the bones of an eighty-year-old.

Someone needed to put all of this information together. I made an appointment with a high-risk OB/GYN because my rheumatologist and regular gynecologist had nothing more to add. They remained of the opinion that pregnancy would be "no problem."

My meeting with the high-risk doctor was somber from the start.

First things first. Without methotrexate I was flaring, and Remicade and prednisone, which I was still on and would likely stay on during pregnancy, weren't doing much to help. This was not a good sign—my body was telling me that it needed the very medication that I would have to stay off while pregnant.

And what about the medication not labeled "Category X"? The data on Remicade and pregnancy is sketchy. There is some data about women who have taken it during their first trimesters, and it appears that their babies all turned out fine.

There is scant information on women who take it any longer, which suggests to me that anyone on Remicade immediately stopped taking it once they knew they were pregnant.

So what if I did stay on Remicade?

"The Remicade might suppress the baby's immune system," the doctor said.

Next we talked bone density.

"Have you broken any bones in unexpected situations?"

Well, yes. At nineteen I broke a bone in my left leg while catching a rebound during an easygoing game of pickup basketball that pitted me against two girls who both hovered around five feet tall. One of them was wearing her shower flip-flops. This was not high-risk behavior, but it still resulted in a bone break, and it took me six months to recover, much longer than expected.

When I was twenty-nine a jumping jack ended with a quiet crack—a stress fracture right above my left ankle. It healed, sort of, but still aches when it rains or I carry piles of heavy books.

I am now prednisone-dependent, so my bone density will only worsen with time. The stress on my hips could trigger a fracture during the pregnancy. Or after. Or maybe even during birth.

Even ignoring all of the above, there was still the unavoidable fact that my pregnancy would be high risk. Something else would go wrong—a third trimester miscarriage or even a stillbirth.

"So, this is what I need to know," I told the doctor, who had neatly parted white hair and seemed willing to give me concrete information.

"What do you recommend?"

He sighed.

"You want me to tell you if you should try to get pregnant?"

"Yes," I nodded.

"I can't. That all depends on your tolerance for risk. You have to make up your own mind. Some women will do anything to have a baby. None of this would stop them. But most women haven't been through what you have."

I nodded some more. My left shoulder began to twitch.

"Let me put it this way, would you fly into Jerusalem tomorrow?"

The week we visited this doctor, the news was filled with stories of air strikes. Most flights in and out of Israeli airports were grounded.

"Well, no, of course not," I said.

"There you have it," the doctor concluded.

He started to close the files on his desk. He wouldn't look me in the eye. He was easing out of his chair, reading to move on to the next appointment.

One foot out the door, he looked back in the room, and suggested surrogacy.

"Well, I don't think I want to pass on my crap genes to anyone else," I told him.

"Adoption's fine," I said.

"I have three adopted daughters," the doctor confessed. "We had fertility issues."

I held it together until I reached the elevator bank, and only then did I let myself cry. Big salty tears dripped down my flushed cheeks. My husband drove me to a bar, the only place I wanted to go, where I scarfed down a hamburger and multiple pink cocktails. I wanted numbness, which is a feeling I never really get to have. I transition from one type of pain to another.

For the next few weeks I'd think I was okay, and then I'd wake up in the middle of the night, remember what I'd learned, and cry some more. I felt like I'd let my husband down—we'd gotten married for many reasons, including that we wanted to have children together. His genes are worth passing on.

But for now we're not going to risk it. In the last five years I've endured two glaucoma surgeries, two ER visits, a pinched nerve, countless knee aspirations and injections, and never-ending physical therapy. Each of these medical events was supposed to be simple but ended up with unpredictable complications and a prolonged recovery.

Even without a baby I'm an unhealthy mess. So we're looking into adoption. And fighting desperately to get me out of this flare. The flare that I walked right into, like an idiot, to see what my body's reaction to getting ready for pregnancy would look like.

I cry less these days. But I do have the lingering memory of a dream in which I saw a young girl, about five years old. She's standing in a field, trying to decide if she should walk through an open wooden gate, the kind with a metal latch that swings back and forth. The grass is high and reaches the bottom of her knee-length dress. Her hair is blonde and cut into a chin-skimming bob—just like mine was at that age.

In my dream she smiles when she sees me and reaches out a small hand, meant for me to fold into one of my own. She's my daughter. I know her. I know her name, too. Jane. Jane like Jane Eyre. Jane so I could call her Janie. Jane, who would be strong and smart and beloved.

I try to push self-pitying moments like this one away. I haven't lost anyone I've held in my arms or carried in my belly. But I lost something.

Maybe it's just the promise of that dream, which I mourn in my own way—quietly, as I muffle my nighttime sobs. I mourn the one I'll never know.

# Reluctant Reliance

ERIN M. KELLY

I woke to the sight of a dull-orange morning sun bleeding through my bedroom window, stirred under my covers for a moment, then noticed an eerie quietness upstairs.

I waited for some all-too-familiar sounds: the soles of shoes making their way down the wooden stairs, the jingling of car keys, a hand on the doorknob of my handicap-accessible entrance.

Silence.

I must have slept through the parade of early morning footsteps. My dad had already left for work, my younger brother for school. There was no click-clank of dishes upstairs in the kitchen either, so I assumed my mom was running her usual morning errands.

I turned my head to find my wheelchair parked in the same spot as it was the night before. It's always parked close to the wall so that the cord from the charger reaches the outlet. The low hum of its motor died down during the night.

The only sounds were my dog, snoring away under my bed, and the roar of cars zipping by on the highway. Just as I was wiping sleep from my eyes, Mother Nature called.

I instinctively reached for my phone, expecting it to be in its usual spot beside my pillow. Nope. I squirmed to the edge of my bed, just enough to peek over the guardrail, to find the phone on the floor.

I didn't know how it got there and I didn't care. I needed that phone in order to do something that most consider simple and second nature. I reminded myself nothing is a "simple" case of mind over matter when a disability is involved.

My cerebral palsy has forced me to rely on my family so much, to the point that I can tell who's coming and going by the sound and rhythm of their footsteps. I've also come to rely on the placement and timing of certain things, as well as the sounds that accompany them. When all of those things seemed nonexistent on this particular morning, my conscience became my only ally. I knew it was the one thing that wasn't going to fail me, even though it was giving me a beat down. I had two choices at this point—yell as loud as I could to see if someone was actually in the house or wait it out and hope for the best. My mind struggled to figure out ways to miraculously fish the phone through the guardrail.

I wanted nothing more than to jump out of my bed, grab my phone, and text someone as fast as my fingers would allow. As with so many other scenarios like this, my cerebral palsy didn't present me with that option.

I didn't mind having to lie in bed. That's a kind of pressure and frustration I've grown accustomed to, but I had extra physical pressure to contend with this morning. That completely changed the game.

Rolled to my right, then left, then to my back. I even rolled on my stomach, but no movement I made was quick or sharp enough to relieve the pressure on my bladder. It only seemed to intensify. I couldn't do a single, solitary thing to help myself. I was physically and mentally exhausted.

And then I heard the sound of my mom's van pulling in the driveway.

"Am I too late?" she asked over the rustling grocery bags.

As I watched her walk into my room and pick up my phone in one smooth, quick motion, I knew this was one of countless incidents in which I've had to surrender to someone else's assistance.

Everyone needs help sometimes, but there's an entirely different level of reliance involved when you have a disability.

After more than thirty years in this role, my mother has a keen awareness of my needs and feelings. It was something she must have sensed when she and my father adopted me as an infant in Korea. I can only imagine what would have happened to me if they hadn't responded to a note that read, "Please adopt to a family that can care for her" upon finding me abandoned in a police station. I've always felt as if that was my parents' promise to me, and they made it knowing they might have a lifetime of challenges ahead of them due to my cerebral palsy.

My mother was not too late. As always, she was right on time.

# An Interview with My Mom

BELINDA WALLER-PETERSON

"I'm glad somebody was interested in my
health or what happened to me in life."
—Valerie Diane Waller

In her book, *I Knew a Woman: The Experience of the Female Body*,
Cortney Davis, nurse practitioner and writer, renders the narratives
of four women who come to her clinic and offers the following:
"When a woman speaks, I catch hold of her words as if they were
silken threads. Slowly I gather them in, braiding the strands and
hoping to create something tangible just by listening."[1] Davis lays
bare what she believes to be a critical and necessary action in the
interaction between patient and caregiver, the sick and the healthy:
*listening* to the story she tells. The act of listening opens a space
for the ill person to reclaim some control over her body by telling
the story of her illness in her own words. The storyteller gives
voice to her own suffering and experience of illness in a way that,
in the moment of telling, liberates her from a dominant medical
narrative that might otherwise seek to impose itself on her and
restrict her articulation of sickness, illness, and the medicalization
of her body. Davis conveys her understanding of this, saying, "and
she did. For thirty minutes, Renee told me her story. The sound
of her voice echoed in the room, bounced around in the hallways
and out into the world, and I was the world, *listening*" (emphasis
mine).[2] The storyteller must be heard. With her permission, this

essay foregrounds the illness narrative of my mother, Valerie Diane Waller. I was tempted to refer to my mother throughout the essay as "Mrs. Waller," but the truth is that this particular piece of writing is deeply personal and I chose to write about her because of our intimate relationship. And, perhaps even more importantly, I need her to be able to see and recognize herself as an individual in my writing, not as a medical subject. She is my mother: her story and her voice matter. I engage the illness narrative tropes of triumph and restitution to explore aspects of my interview with my mother and retell her story of asthma's impact on her life. This essay presents her story in two parts: *Beginnings* and *Learning to Live Again*.

My mom was sixty-one years old in 2012 when we sat down in the front room of my house to talk about her experience with asthma. I interviewed her as part of an illness narrative project. Our interview provided me the opportunity to hear her tell a familiar story, one that we lived through while I was working on my bachelor of science in nursing degree. She developed adult-onset asthma after she was exposed to secondhand smoke in her workplace. What began as bronchitis slowly morphed into wheezing and a persistent cough that lasted a few months. Her doctors diagnosed her with asthma and referred her to specialists. After some trial and error, her doctors discovered a therapeutic regimen that managed the condition and restored her quality of life. That is the bare bones of what happened to my mom, some version of which might exist in her medical records. However, her illness narrative conveys the crucial role she played in recovering her health, which in addition to her changed mental and physical health includes overcoming the challenges, skepticism, and shunning she encountered from co-workers, family, and friends. While I had background knowledge of her condition and some of the experiences that occurred, this interview allowed me to hear the story from her unique perspective and revealed previously unknown details, some of which were difficult to hear. At one point my mom said, "But yes, so, . . . that's my stuff. And I saw the tears and waters in your eyes." I did not expect to have such an emotional response to my mother's story because of our previous conversations, yet I found myself feeling a range of emotions, especially when she wove me into her narrative. She allowed me to see myself anew in the moments she described, and I relived those feelings of helplessness and confusion when I watched my mother's body, in various hospital beds, tormented with relentless fits of coughing. We cried and laughed together as she told her story, and in the end I was physically and emotionally spent as if I were the one who had endured the struggle; but I was the listener and this was her story.

## I. Beginnings

Even before the official diagnosis, bronchitis greatly impacted my mom's life. She describes "walking around with a nagging cough," feeling as if she could not breathe, and "not being able to do the things" she used to be able to do. For months she attempted to follow her usual routines, only to find that her changed body was now hypersensitive to smells and would, without warning, restrict her airways and send her into sustained coughing spells that ended with her feeling physically exhausted. Her condition was exacerbated by her "work situation" that consisted of moldy smells and people smoking in and out of the office; she says,

> I would say that was a big impact because on a daily base when you're going to work, thinking you're going to be able to work, and no you get there and . . . then you would have a person that opens their office door and the smoke just hits you okay, and you try to explain to them that no your doctor said you need to be away from the smoke . . .

Despite the frequent visits to the emergency room and doctor's office because of the attacks, conditions at my mom's job remained unchanged. Some of her more inconsiderate co-workers continued to smoke right outside of the building near the door and in some cases behind the closed doors of their offices. She was encouraged by her more compassionate co-workers to go outside and get some fresh air after her attacks. However, even this suggestion contributed to additional episodes as she encountered the trigger again upon her return to her desk. She experienced attacks sometimes twice a day and three times a week. My mom gave a shocking example of how she was treated at work saying,

> They moved my . . . desk in front of her office [the woman who was smoking] . . . and she was actually my supervisor and I said to her, no, I can't sit here because every time you open your door that smell comes out . . . and then you wanna have meetings in your office and I can't come into your office. So I talked to human resource . . . so what we, what *they* came up with, it's okay that she smokes in her office . . . and I had it all in writing . . . I have everything, emails through, saying what was going on, and so she said, no it's okay she smokes in her office and long as her door is closed, and the hours you are there from 8–12, . . . she can, . . . long as you're not there she is able to smoke. I said you don't understand, when she opens that door that smoke stuff lingers.

Her supervisor's and Human Resources' refusal to change or enforce workplace practices related to smoking regulations promoted a culture of misunderstanding about asthma, its triggers, and the responsibility of businesses in protecting the health and well-being of their employees. Rather than using my mom's condition as an opportunity to educate employees, her employer attempted to intimidate and punish her for speaking up for herself and demanding a smoke-free work environment. She continues,

> So, with all that in mind, you know, that, that made my lungs weaker . . . at that point, so that's when all these other scents,

like strong perfumes . . . and um, cleaning chemicals, you know because your system is already weak . . . and then those things started setting it off as well, you know, so (pause) to me it was a really big impact because people would go, "well I can wear perfume if I want" [My mom uses a nasty tone to represent these people]. Yes, you have the right to wear perfume, I'm not saying you don't . . . stay away from me with your perfume!"

She laughed when she said this, I suspect because of the absurdity associated with someone insisting that their right to smell good superseded her right to breathe. The point becomes even more ridiculous for her as she notes throughout her story that all she wants is to be able to go through her day without having an asthma attack that causes her to wet herself and end up in the emergency room receiving breathing treatments. The disruption this particular illness created in my mom's life manifested in ways that her co-workers and supervisor could not relate to or even begin to process. As a result, her condition deteriorated to include sensitivity to perfumes and cleaning products, which ultimately shrank the size of her world and limited her social mobility. Instead of being able to shop at Macy's, attend church and school, go to work, have lunch with friends, or even clean the house, she felt weakened, shunned, and confined to her house.

The frequency of the attacks and their exhaustive nature impacted my mom beyond the workplace, which was especially difficult for her because she has always been fiercely independent and incredibly productive in all aspects of her life. She was working on her undergraduate degree in accounting when the illness began, and as a result of the bronchitis, the hacking cough, and the all of the doctor's appointments, her grades began to slip. Her inability to study and perform well in school fueled her frustration about her doctor's failure to manage the illness so that she could go back to living her life. Ultimately, the severity and unpredictability of the attacks forced her to work and attend school from home. She did this for two and half years. My mom spent very little time speaking about her grades. Instead she laughed and said, "Oh, this is not fair! You know," then went back to talking about how she spoke out against the job's discriminatory work practices. Even though my mom spoke in great detail about the trials of working in an office with people that did not care about her health and seemed to go out of their way to aggravate her condition, she did so with a smile on her face and a knowing tone that led me to understand that this story would end in her favor. She moved through the telling of her initial bout with asthma in a way that balanced the many ordeals with the hard-earned triumphs.

## II. Learning to Live Again

So much of my mom's story details her struggle to prove that what she experienced was real and to claim her illness in the public spaces that she was expected to navigate (work, church). She repeatedly described the way that co-workers, family, and friends would antagonize her and accuse her of making up or causing her own attacks.

She constructed her narrative to highlight the obstacles that she overcame, including an attack that resulted in rescue emergency coming to her job to take her to the hospital; an attack in the hospital as a result of her nurse wearing perfume that confirmed her illness; a hospitalization as a result of a medication transcription error that almost killed her; and her self-tapering of her medication. She conveyed her sense of her illness through the gaze of someone fighting against the odds in order regain her life, pre-asthma. That movement toward reclamation could only begin with the acknowledgment that her illness was not constructed, imagined, or in any other way mediated by my mom.

Two stories exemplify moments when all of my mom's attacks were validated and she seized control of her medical treatment: first, the story of an attack during her hospitalization; and second, her self-tapering her medication. Before I retell those stories, I want to briefly acknowledge the moment when her doctor finally discovered a medication that effectively worked against her asthma, which ultimately led to her freedom from hospitalizations, breathing treatments, inhalers, and a litany of medications. My mom reports that after one of her treatments in her doctor's office "when he actually came in to check after the treatment, he goes, 'wait a minute, wait a minute,' [excitement in her voice]. 'I think we might've finally found a breakthrough. You do have asthma. You really, really do have asthma.'" This helped to redefine the ways in which she thought about her illness and seemed to shape her determination to overcome asthma.

*Story One*: After one of her more serious attacks at work, my mom was admitted to the hospital for a week where she was monitored and her doctor continued to try different medications to manage her asthma. She recalls,

> When I got released from the hospital, the nurse that wrote the prescription (pause) . . . overmedicated me 'cause she doubled the . . . the medication . . . and whatever, and that's why y'all got a call saying mom is in the ER and I had to drink the charcoal . . . to live (pause) because I had poison in my bloodstream . . . . . . and whatever, oh yea. I went through.

As my mom begins this story, I can also remember receiving the phone call from my dad to come down to the hospital right away because she was not well. The call was alarming and disconcerting because my dad, who was typically even-handed and calm (he was a Marine for twenty-three years), was noticeably upset. This is the point in her narrative where I can feel the tears burning my eyes. Her words echo in my ears,

> I took those [pills], and when I took them, you know, I had so much energy. . . . 'cause first I was so tired when I went home,

and then I had so much energy. And I'm getting up 2 o'clock in the morning, telling dad I'm starving . . . it's like I was, it was on drugs, okay. I'm starving . . . I went down and I fixed a full breakfast, like potatoes . . . the whole works, okay, and then dad goes, and, and he, he didn't even tell me what he suspect was going on. He called the hospital that Sunday morning and talked to them and what he said I don't know, (laughs), okay, but he said, I'll be right back, I've gotta run around the corner but if they call, just tell me what they say . . . you know. . . . So, when he came back he said, um, we're going to um, um, the hospital actually called and they want me to bring you in, and everything. He never told me what the suspicious was, okay. So I got dressed and we went, you know, and everything, and um, so I got re-hospitalized.

. . . and in the process of them, um, giving me the charcoal . . . they wanted me to stay overnight cause they wanted to monitor my heart rate . . . to make sure I wasn't gonna have a cardiac arrest. Okay, which, that was a fear for everybody at that point but to me, . . . and then they tell me, . . . you got um, blood poisoning, . . . you have medication too much in you, it's poisoning your blood, and I goes, okay, well whatever you have to do, you know . . .

And to me, *drinking* the, . . . the grit of charcoal, and I knew it was serious when dad's calling pastor during the time I'm there and it's during morning service, and, and everything, and he comes afterwards and "oh, let's have prayer" you know, I'm like . . . whoa, what is going on . . . I still didn't realize how bad off I was . . . okay, because I didn't, I didn't feel, I just felt like I was on a cloud somewhere, you know. I just got all this energy.

I realized, . . . when they kept saying, no you have to drink the charcoal, you have to, and that's the only way we can get it out. And I, I can't remember if they had another solution, but that was the one that they really wanted to use, was the charcoal. And that they said no, . . . and that's why your dad called all of y'all, you and Reggie, . . . and then when I . . . seen y'all coming to the hospital, I think that's when I really realized for sure, that oh am I gonna die today? (laughs)

And then I realized the next morning when I woke up . . . in the morning and um, shortly after I had waken up, my mom was there again, you know, 'cause she had came to visit me. All of them came down when I was in for the week . . . but . . . when dad told her Sunday I was in, she came first thing Monday morning. And she was there while he was there too, and then all of a sudden pastor pops up, "oh, you look 360 degrees better than you did yesterday" (laughs). And, . . . I really felt blessed at that point.

And then, it was funny because I was sitting there talking to my mom, I was sitting there on the bed facing . . . that little auditorium [with her back to the door], . . . and as I was sitting there . . . the nurse that had been in earlier that day came back, . . . and I didn't see her when she came in, okay, but when she came in something sparked, something she had on sparked an attack . . . but then when she said what happened, . . . I said, no I know you was here earlier, I don't know what the difference is. And she said I can almost tell you. I said I *smell* something, you know . . . and I can still smell it and I had the attack . . . with my back to her not knowing she was there, . . . one of the patients had gave her some perfume . . . and she put it on. And she said Oh my gosh, I'm never gonna do this again, and whatever. And see, . . . at a point, psychologically, people was thinking that's what was happening . . . I'm just doing this for attention. Because . . . I even took a test so that they know I'm not playing with this (laughs).

Overmedicated, charcoal to live, poison in her bloodstream . . . my mom lay on that hospital bed fighting to regain her body and hold onto her life. Completely unaware of how precarious her condition was, my mom struggled to make sense of this newest crisis related to her asthma. It was heart-wrenching to hear her talk about how she was absolutely disconnected from the reality of the moment until her pastor, mother, and children all arrived at the hospital. This was also the first time that I heard her talk so candidly about the prospect of dying that day. Even a decade and a half later, she recalled the episode with great clarity, detail, and emotion.

One of the main points my mom made throughout her interview was that she refused to be a victim and struggled against people's insensitivity about and disbelief of her illness. The story of the nurse and her perfume is especially triumphant for my mom because the mid-shift change serves as an undeniable before-and-after case study. Up to this point, certain people believed that she was faking her illness. However, the nurse revealed that she was not wearing any perfume earlier in the morning when she saw my mom but since that time had been given perfume as a gift from another patient. The nurse tried it on and continued caring for her patients. When she returned to my mom's room the perfume caused her to have an asthma attack. In this moment my mom believed she was finally vindicated; she had witnesses and her illness was confirmed.

My mom was also very forthcoming in other areas regarding her struggle with asthma. When asked to talk about her feelings about her doctor and how she was treated as a patient she did not hesitate to say that he "was pretty good for the most part" but there "would be times, when he would . . . really tick me off." She believes that he thought she was "agitating something" up until the moment he realized the newest asthma medication he tried with her worked and claims that she was able to see "the real side of him when he was able to make a breakthrough one day, with the medication." My mom does not portray her doctor as a saint, savior, or a *complete* hindrance to her recovery process. He was someone who tried to find different medications to help alleviate and relieve her asthma attacks yet had a grave misunderstanding of her illness trajectory (he expected her to be on asthma medication for the rest of her life). This last point is one that she identifies as the moment that caused her to change her lifestyle. To this end she tapered her medication without her doctor's approval. The break that she makes from her doctor's prescribed medical path signals a clear push back against the medicalization of her body *and* her refusal to be "written on from the outside."[3]

*Story Two*: My mom reclaimed her lost voice by reducing the amount of medication she took until she was not taking any at all. She says, "so, actually what I did is, and I know it wasn't right, or whatever, but what I did was I weaned myself off everyday . . . off the medication. Because I knew that I did not need to." And she reports that when she went to his office for a breathing treatment, he told her that her numbers were "looking good," to which she replied,

> "Hmmm, interesting, 'cause I have to confess, I have, you know, not taken any medication . . . or anything, for the past month and a half . . . and I said, I understand what I did . . . but I did it on a gradual base. I said, and I told my husband exactly what I was gonna do . . . and I always had my emergency inhaler."

She challenged the medical expertise of her doctor that seeks to inscribe illness on her body for the rest of her life. Faced with the prospect of staying on medication for the rest of her life, and after years of struggling with the stigma of asthma and failed treatments, she determined to control her own body.

## Conclusion

My mom is a wounded storyteller who deeply values her illness narrative.[4] She was excited to talk about how she triumphed over asthma through perseverance and self-discipline and was quick to characterize it as an ordeal she went through *in her past*. She details specific practices that helped her to overcome her illness, including exercise and a personal commitment to well-being. She presents her narrative as a triumphant one and, while she readily admits that there is always a possibility that her asthma will return, she lives her life free from its restraints. When reflecting on the negative ways that asthma impacted her life, my mom said that her illness "stopped me from being able to go to restaurants, being able to do those things. So, that's why . . . I feel like I have my freedom back." When asked what lesson she learned from her experience with asthma she responded with the following:

> The one thing I would take away is no, . . . no, you do not have to do this [work someplace where the conditions are not in your best interest]. And it wasn't like I was in a financial bind, and that's what I'll tell people over and over now. That a lot of times things happen because jobs think they got you over, then they gonna do that . . . so um, that's my whole thing. You got to cover your own.

She expressed her new understanding of illness through the eyes of a belligerent society—in this case her workplace formed the core of this society. She cautioned others to recognize their own value even when others attempt to lull them into accepting substandard conditions that negatively impact their health and life. This lesson informed her narrative. She invested in telling her story in a way that detailed her most difficult struggles against asthma, her job, and at times, her doctors. My mom's desire to control her story and take action against her illness, even against medical orders, demonstrates the importance of self-determination in the face of sickness. She explicitly states that she knew better than her doctor what her body needed and what the outcome of her illness would be. She goes on to reclaim her body and victory over her illness, despite the odds against her, her insensitive co-workers, fellow church members, and family. Her story is one that demonstrates successful reclamation of agency over one's body. She stands on the other side of her illness, primarily in the land of the healthy, and names asthma as something that is in her past; "and that's my stuff" she says. "I'm glad somebody was interested in my health or what happened to me in life."

## Notes

1. Cortney Davis, *I Knew a Woman: The Experience of the Female Body* (New York: Random House, 2001), 183.
2. Davis, *I Knew a Woman*, 185.
3. Arthur Frank, *The Wounded Storyteller: Body, Illness, and Ethics* (Chicago: University of Chicago Press, 1995), 71.
4. Frank defines a wounded storyteller as someone who has experiences and tells the story of his or her illness.

# Days of the Giants

MADALINE HARRISON

Days of the giants. When I was in training the attendings used that phrase, often after telling a story from earlier days in medicine, describing a harrowing night on call or a now legendary professor who could pull a diagnosis out of his hat like a rabbit. *I was there*, the phrase implied, a sign like a secret handshake.

I have just indulged in such an anecdote. As the team continues through the hospital on morning rounds, I can see the residents mentally roll their eyes and imagine they are thinking *"dinosaurs"* or something less polite. For a moment I imagine myself tilting at windmills, riding a swaybacked, spavined charger across the plain toward an illusory enemy—defending a vanishing tradition.

We move to the next room. There is no shortage of real enemies here and elsewhere: war, famine, pestilence, and death. We concern ourselves in the hospital mostly with the last two. As the residents dip and hover over their tiny screens, I look past them down the years to a corridor of hospital rooms or, earlier still, into a wide room filled with curtained alcoves, each one containing a stretcher.

Medicine still contains an oral tradition, passed down in stories: the stories patients tell us, the ones we tell them and the ones we tell ourselves. There is also the story of medicine, Medicine with a capital *M*, the history we place ourselves in as we construct our own narratives of becoming physicians. The names of early physicians, embedded in the names of diseases or now obscure signs used in physical diagnosis, hint at that history: Friedreich's ataxia, the Babinski sign. My own field, neurology, is particularly notorious for eponyms. There are hundreds of them. Today advances in technology allow us the illusion that we can see what is hidden, no longer depending solely on our eyes and ears, just as sailors no longer rely on scanning the waves to detect a change in the current or the subtle difference in the color of the water that signals a sandbar. But the doctors before us did, and their stories echo in the names we use for the diseases they defined.

When I talk about Huntington's disease, I like to tell the story of George Huntington, making rounds with his father and grandfather by buggy, returning later to study the disease that devastated those families on Long Island. We know now that his ancestors and those of the families he described came over from East Anglia in the same fleet, their stories now permanently joined. I think of the Huntington's families I have known, pedigrees stretching over pages and across the boundaries we place between ourselves and illness. I have a high school friend whose mother's cousin I have followed for years, although she does not know and I cannot tell her. A family who lived just a mile from me found their way to the Huntington's clinic. My patient danced every Friday at the free concert, his uncontrolled choreic movements submerged in the dance. I passed his wife on the road and at back-to-school night, always alone.

I did not start out intending to become a doctor. I graduated from college in the 1970s with a degree in psychology. It was a time filled with uncertainty. Unemployment was high and gas was rationed. In a borrowed car, an old turquoise Studebaker with one cement fender, I arrived at the local mental health clinic to interview for a federally funded position as a psychiatric emergency services coordinator. Not many college graduates showed up for those interviews, and they hired me on the spot. The regional administrator and the psychiatrist who ran the clinic shared space on the third floor of a small local hospital, and when the funds ran out, I stayed on at the clinic as a counselor.

There are a few stories I find myself telling from those days. During my first week on the job I made the rounds, introducing myself to the local agencies. One of my first stops was the state psychiatric hospital, a complex of towering Gothic brick buildings right out of a Hollywood set. The administrative offices lined a cavernous hallway paneled in dark wood. While I waited on a bench outside the nursing director's office, a tiny woman approached me and asked for matches. I already knew enough to know the answer to *that* question, but I did offer to light the cigarette she was holding. She inhaled deeply, blew the smoke out close to my head, and said, "I wish I could get this woman out of my body." I don't remember what, or if, I answered.

I made home visits with the clinic psychiatrist to see a woman who had not left her house in years, except for occasional forays to find a doctor who would amputate the contaminated toe that drove her to spend hours each day relentlessly scrubbing herself and the house. Another time, I accompanied the small-town police on a psychiatric emergency call and watched as they retrieved a terrified exchange student from the closet where he had been hiding for three days. After we arrived at the state hospital, I pushed the button to close the elevator doors, watching five attendants struggle to hold him as he fought, convinced that the doors were closing on a gas chamber. I could never have imagined such afflictions.

Later, as a medical student, I was intoxicated by the panorama of science, enchanted by the glowing console of the electron microscope, like the control panel of a spaceship exploring the smallest imaginable spaces. I marveled at the neuroanatomy professor who could draw the brain or spinal cord two-handed, the outline appearing from under his chalk like a butterfly. I was astonished by the intricate machinery of the body and the infinite variety of ways in which things could go wrong. But it was in the hospital that I became a doctor.

As a second-year medical student I went to the VA Hospital

with two classmates every Tuesday afternoon for physical diagnosis rounds. Our preceptor was a renowned specialist in diseases of the liver, a useful skill in a hospital filled with every possible consequence of alcoholism. He must have been close to eighty at the time I knew him. We would start each session in his office, and I watched my fellow students roll their eyes or nudge each other while he talked. I knew from their comments as we walked over that they thought he was a doddering has-been, an old man rambling on. And perhaps he was. I don't remember now what he would say in those sessions. But I will never forget watching him in the hospital.

We would enter the ward, rows of beds lining the sides of the large room. Without hesitation he would stride toward the nearest occupied bed, knowing nothing about the man sitting or lying there, or his illness. After a handshake he would draw out the outlines of each story in a few questions, followed by a respectful approach to the problem area, including us in the laying on of hands. Many of those men faced an uncertain fate, but we left them reassured, at least for the moment, by the doctor's interest and the certainty he conveyed that, whatever the outcome, their doctors were good ones and were doing their best to help. Week after week I watched him work that same magic and tried to uncover how he did it, the hidden panel in the floor of the safe or the back of the box. But, as I gradually understood, there was no trick. He cared about those men, and all the others like them he had cared for, and knew the power of hope when there was little else to offer.

The following year I began my work in the hospital as a clinical clerk, rotating from one part of the hospital to another to learn about the various branches of medicine. This was the work for which those sessions at the va were to have prepared me. My time was divided between Jackson Memorial Hospital and the va Jackson Memorial Hospital in the 1980s was a war zone. By now similar stories have been told in any number of TV medical dramas, but to a student there was nothing of the cliché about it. In those days Jackson was a sprawling complex dominated by a fourteen-story tower that was surrounded by low buildings housing the older wards and the emergency room. An endless polyglot stream of patients flowed in from all over Miami and beyond. Miami itself was filled with immigrants from Latin America and the Caribbean, and more arrived daily. They came from Cuban jails on the Mariel boatlift or floated over from Haiti on makeshift rafts. The sickest came straight from the docks to the Jackson emergency room.

With little in the way of preliminaries, the students were thrown into this teeming mix and expected to put their hand to whatever task most urgently required attention—starting an IV, sewing up a laceration, drawing a blood gas, pushing a patient to X-ray, or running a tube of blood to the lab. We struggled to complete the items on the "scut" list. On surgery we trailed the teams, the pockets of our short white coats stuffed with gauze and tape, hurrying to catch up after changing a dressing. The trauma service overflowed with GSWs, young men admitted with gunshot wounds, shackled to the bed with handcuffs to receive our ministrations. The surgeons worked shifts unimaginable now, thirty-six hours on, twelve off if that. Even after the on-call team came on, they lingered around the nurses' stations, laughing and telling stories.

The pediatric surgery service was legendary for the skill and dedication of the attendings. I signed up for two weeks, although I was not interested in either pediatrics or surgery as a career. I watched as they bent over their tiny patients, some barely bigger than the hands of the six-foot four-inch attending, with what seemed to be infinite patience and tenderness. The fellow had already completed a full surgical training in Brazil. Ironic, with a hollow face and ageless eyes, he admonished the students. "Hurry up," he'd say as we wrapped up the day's work, "I must get home—my kids are crying." But I'd see him later, stopping by once again to check on a sick infant before he made his way home.

Upstairs on the obstetrics floor chaos reigned as women arrived in every conceivable stage of labor, delivering in the elevator or the prep room, flying down the hallways to the delivery room on stretchers, the OB teams calling out, "Primip on the table!", primiparous referring to a first-time mother. On the maternity wards the halls were lined with stretchers cordoned off with portable curtains as the deliveries approached ten thousand that year. We learned *push/don't push* in Spanish and Creole and took turns "catching" the slippery newborns.

On the medicine wards, among the uncontrolled diabetics and the asthmatics struggling for breath, a growing number of patients were arriving with a puzzling set of complaints: Haitians with intractable diarrhea, a persistent cough, and weight loss; young gay men with strange purple splotches, sudden crises of fever, and rapid collapse. At night the ward was filled with faint ghostly coughing. In those days we didn't wear gloves to draw blood or start IVs, but when a young Haitian woman was admitted a resident took me aside and warned me to wear gloves this time. It was another year before this disease had a name and even longer before such precautions became routine.

The emergency room was the filter through which this flood of humanity had to pass under the watchful eyes of the Miami–Dade County police. Teams of battle-hardened doctors and nurses triaged the patients in order of urgency, directly to the trauma bay or cardiac suite, or into the tank of insecticide for delousing. One veteran nurse wore a Barnum and Bailey button on his scrubs, proclaiming this "The Greatest Show on Earth." On the wall was a bulletin board with a line of cockroaches pulled from ear canals and neatly skewered with hypodermic tips, next to a worn piece of paper on which a key to Cuban prison tattoos was printed. In the parking lot behind the ER stood rows of refrigerated trailers belonging to the medical examiner's office. In the ER I performed my first spinal tap, the intern narrating my instructions as if speak-

ing to the patient, an elderly black man who lay on a stretcher, a
sheet holding his knees in place.

"You'll feel a little pinch as we put in the anesthetic . . ." and so
on until we were done. It went well and the intern was so pleased
that once we had finished he hurried around to the front of the
stretcher and congratulated the patient.

"You are a lucky man," he said. "That doctor has golden hands."
The patient stared.

"You mean you let a *woman* put that needle in my back?" The
intern laughed and clapped the patient on the shoulder, and we
headed upstairs.

As students we were often the only members of the medical team
who saw the patient for much of the time, the interns and residents
busy with newer or sicker patients. It went without saying that it
was up to us to get the job done, whatever it was. In the face of this
the students banded together, trading insider knowledge: tips for
tying a surgeon's knot, for finding a vein, or for getting along with
this or that attending. We watched in awe at morning report as
the seasoned interns presented their admissions, reciting labs from
memory which were, if not identical, at least close to the actual
values, and confidently reeling off a list of increasingly esoteric
possibilities in the differential diagnosis.

The patients looked to us for help, for explanations, for reassur-
ance. There were few translators available, one of the consequences
of a law passed prohibiting the use of county funds to promote
any language other than English. I got better at patching together
a hybrid medical Spanish, often trying out the medical term with
what I hoped was a passable Spanish pronunciation: "Bomi*tare*?
Tachycardi*a*?"

I returned to Jackson Memorial for my internship. The resident,
a gruff Cuban woman who had been one of the toughest, most
respected interns, met me when I arrived at 7:00 that morning.

"Your first admission is in the emergency room," she said, sending me off with a list of the other patients I was assigned.

I arrived and was sent over to a corner of the holding area where patients awaiting admission were lined up on stretchers. My patient was a thin black man in his fifties, with blood pressure so high it had caused swelling in his brain and bleeding at the back of his eyes. He was one of the few judged sick enough to require ICU admission, but until then my job was to sit by the stretcher and take his blood pressure every ten minutes as medication was dripped in through an IV to lower his blood pressure enough but not so much that he would suffer a stroke. Seven hours later a nurse stopped by to tell me that the MICU had a bed for him, only to return a few minutes later with the news that the bed had gone to someone else. Numb with despair I resumed my task, dutifully pumping up and releasing the cuff, adding to the column of numbers on the clipboard by the stretcher. Three hours later the resident arrived just as the orderlies showed up to take my patient to the unit. She handed me a sign-out sheet with the names of my next five admissions and the other interns' patients for whom I was responsible overnight. With a brisk "See you in the morning," she was gone.

At that time the on-call interns handled new patients from the emergency room until midnight, often taking on two to three more in a frantic countdown between 11:00 and midnight. Through the rest of the night we "worked them up", asking our questions, listening to heart and lungs, reviewing their hospital charts, wheeling them to X-ray, starting their IVs, and drawing blood. This was before electronic medical records and a world away from hospitals with IV nurses or even transportation aides, at least after midnight. The charts were piled in stacks like telephone books, the X-rays in slippery piles behind counters in the darkened film room. Once the work was completed, the patients "tucked in," we sat down to write up each admission, and with any luck had time for a shower or breakfast before rounds the next morning. My last chore after each on-call night was to stop by the ward to check on my patients and enter any remaining lab values in my writeup. Often I would find them already filled in, the attending having gotten there before me.

But even he did not accompany me to Ward D, the prison ward. Once morning rounds were completed I would make my way to the concrete corridor that led to the entrance, marked by a sign that admonished "Do Not Loiter in This Area." The guard buzzed me through the door and, once it closed behind me, buzzed again to admit me to the ward from the entryway, windows reinforced with wire mesh. I had one patient there, an IV drug user being treated for a heart infection caused by bacteria from contaminated needles. He was getting worse. The nurses called and I came, but I did not know what else to do beyond the drugs he was already getting. He was scared and so was I.

One night on call, I told the cross-cover resident about him. "Would you like me to go see him with you?" he asked. There was nothing I wanted more. Within minutes the resident was on the phone arranging emergency surgery to remove the irretrievably damaged valves in my patient's heart, but he never returned from the operating room.

I don't tell that story on rounds, but I often think of it. There are other stories after I had learned what to do and, with varying combinations of skill and luck, brought my patients through, at least that time. And other times when there was nothing anyone could have done. There were moments of comedy, the black humor variety now frowned on. "Did I ever tell you about the time I was almost peed on by a leper?" True story. I don't tell that one on rounds either, although sometimes I imagine the startled looks I would get, the residents lifting their heads in surprise from the flickering screens.

For better or worse, that is the tradition to which I belong. And it was as often worse as better—exhausted young doctors doing an impossible job, but pulling it off more often than not, night after night. We learned the hard way and paid a price, as did our patients.

I am not sure when in the course of this sometimes-brutal initiation I began to listen differently, to hear the other stories. In the CCU I took care of an Israeli pianist after he had a heart attack. I don't remember now which coronary artery was involved. I don't remember whether he had heart failure or not. I do remember he survived, as he had before. As I had been trained to do, I took a history—when the chest pain started, nausea or not, shortness of breath or not. And then I got to the arm—not the one he had, but the one that was missing. His wife was sitting next to him as I ran through my questions. It was impossible not to notice that she too was missing an arm. I asked and they told me. Before the war he was a pianist and she was a violinist. In the camp each had an arm amputated, to prevent them from continuing their music. They survived and after the war, they settled in Israel. He learned to play one-handed and she became a singer. They toured in Israel and in Europe, performing the music of their survival and songs for those who did not survive.

Not all the stories span an epoch in history or the full eight octaves that the human spirit contains. Sometimes it is a simple detail—the time that my patient took off for a West Virginia bar on the riding mower before Huntington's disease confined him to a wheelchair, or the name of the parakeet that fills my ataxic patient's housebound world. One day, going through my mail, I opened an envelope and out fell a picture of my patient, the parakeet sitting on her head.

Remembering these and so many other stories, what I feel now is compassion: for my patients, for myself as a young doctor, and for the students and residents coming behind me. Their world is different. A thin veil of protocols and policies is draped over the rawness and chaos of injury and illness. The residents clock in and clock out, tracking "duty hours" at the behest of a huge bureaucracy that looms behind the scenes, ready to impose sanctions on any program whose residents spend an additional unauthorized hour caring for their patients. There are elaborate procedures to pass on information among the rotating teams of doctors who are caring for patients they haven't met before and won't see again. Residents log in the supervised procedures they must perform before being authorized to attempt them on their own and complete required computer modules on everything from hand-washing technique to the protocol to be followed in the event of a bomb threat.

And yet there is much that hasn't changed, as I am learning still— from my patients but also from the young doctors I am charged with teaching. A third-year medical student, new to the hospital as I was once, stayed behind after rounds and stood with a family as their twenty- year-old son was declared brain-dead. At their request she stayed with him while he was extubated. An intern returned after her shift to the bedside of a young man wracked with uncontrolled dystonic muscle spasms and held his head to relieve his parents so they could have dinner together. Before she left that night she ordered the medication I had told her wouldn't help, and it didn't. But the next morning I knew she had been there, and why.

Days of the giants? A myth—there are no giants. Or perhaps more of an epic poem than a myth, passed down and changed by each teller as the times change, that links the legendary physicians of the past to the students and residents standing beside me at the door to the next room, where another story is unfolding. I step inside, uncertain what challenge I will find and whether I will be equal to it. I ready myself to listen. The story begins, and I hope for the heart to see it through.

# Source Acknowledgments

Brian Doyle, "Two Hearts," first appeared in *Leaping: Revelations & Epiphanies* (Loyola Press, 2003). Reprinted by permission of the author. © 2017 by Brian Doyle.

Deborah Burghardt, "Spared," © 2017 by Deborah Burghardt.

Floyd Skloot, "A Measure of Acceptance," first appeared in *Creative Nonfiction* 19 (2002). Reprinted by permission of the author. © 2017 by Floyd Skloot.

Matthew S. Smith, "One Little Mind, Our Lie, Dr. Lie," first appeared in *Neurology* 87 (2016): 232–33. Reprinted with permission of the publisher. © 2016 Wolters Klower.

Mark Brazaitis, "Locked into Life," first appeared in *The Sun* 460 (April 2014). Reprinted by permission of the author. © 2017 by Mark Brazaitis.

Teresa Blankmeyer Burke, "Rendered Mute," first appeared in *Atrium* 12 (Winter 2014). Reprinted by permission of the author. © 2017 by Teresa Blankmeyer Burke.

Michael Bérubé, "Jamie's Place," first appeared in *Aeon*, November 1, 2016. Reprinted by permission of the author. © 2016 by Michael Bérubé.

Sonya Huber, "A Day in the Grammar of Disease," first appeared in *Brevity* 43 (May 2013). Reprinted by permission of the author. © 2017 by Sonya Huber.

Source Acknowledgments

William Bradley, "Marked," first appeared in *Cleaver* 8 (December 2014). Reprinted by permission of the author. © 2017 by William Bradley.

Rebecca Housel, "750 Words about Cancer," first appeared in *Brevity* 22 (Fall 2006). Reprinted by permission of the author. © 2017 by Rebecca Housel.

Hugh Silk, "The Power of a Handshake," first appeared in *Intima*, Spring 2015. Reprinted by permission of the author. © 2017 by Hugh Silk.

Tenley Lozano, "Submerged," was the winner of the 2017 John Guyon Literary Nonfiction Prize sponsored by *Crab Orchard Review; Crab Orchard Review* 22 (January 1, 2018). © 2018 by Tenley Lozano.

Kat Moore, "Where Do You Go from Alston Street?" first appeared in *Hippocampus Magazine*, April 1, 2016. Reprinted by permission of the author. © 2017 by Kat Moore.

Diane Kraynak, "Confession," © 2017 by Diane Kraynak.

Adriana Páramo, "This Moment," first appeared in *Brevity* 47 (Fall 2014). Reprinted by permission of the author. © 2017 by Adriana Páramo.

Elizabeth Brady, "Sit Still and Uncover Your Eyes," first appeared in *Modern Loss*, August 13, 2015. Reprinted by permission of the author. © 2017 by Elizabeth Brady.

Meredith Davies Hadaway, "Overtones," © 2017 by Meredith Davies Hadaway.

Patrick Donnelly, "The Way of the Spring," first appeared in the blog Living with Chronic Illness, December 23, 2010. Reprinted by permission of the author. © 2017 by Patrick Donnelly.

Riley Passmore, "Type One," first appeared in *Sweet: A Literary Confection* 8, no. 1. Reprinted by permission of the author. © 2017 by Riley Passmore.

Sandra Beasley, "The Bad Patient," © 2017 by Sandra Beasley.

Taison Bell, "A Tribute to the Pharmacist," first appeared in *MedPage Today's* KevinMD.com, March 24, 2017. Reprinted by permission of the author. © 2017 by Taison Bell.

Katherine MacFarlane, "Flying into Jerusalem," first appeared in *Intima* (Spring 2015). Reprinted by permission of the author. © 2017 by Katherine MacFarlane.

Erin M. Kelly, "Reluctant Reliance," first appeared in *The Huffington Post*, January 21, 2014. Reprinted by permission of the author. © 2017 by Erin M. Kelly.

Belinda Waller-Peterson, "An Interview with My Mom," © 2017 by Belinda Waller-Peterson.

Madaline Harrison, "Days of the Giants," first appeared in *Hospital Drive*, August–September 2015. Reprinted by permission of the author. © 2017 by Madaline Harrison.

# Contributors

SANDRA BEASLEY is the author of *Don't Kill the Birthday Girl: Tales from an Allergic Life,* a memoir and cultural history of food allergies. Her essays and articles have been featured in *The New York Times, Washington Post, Creative Nonfiction, The Oxford American,* and elsewhere. She is also the author of three poetry collections, including *Count the Waves* (W.W. Norton). Honors for her work include a Literature Fellowship from the National Endowment for the Arts and the Maureen Egen Exchange Award from *Poets & Writers.* Beasley lives in Washington DC. She teaches poetry and nonfiction with the University of Tampa low-residency MFA program.

TAISON BELL is an Assistant Professor of Medicine in the divisions of Pulmonary/Critical Care and Infectious Disease at the University of Virginia Medical School. He attended the University of Virginia and graduated with a Bachelor's degree in African American Studies. He then attended medical school at the Columbia College of Physicians and Surgeons, before completing his internship, residency, and ID fellowship at the Massachusetts General Hospital. He then completed his critical care fellowship at the National Institutes of Health. At UVA his work focuses on quality improvement initiatives for critically ill patients.

MICHAEL BÉRUBÉ is an Edwin Erle Sparks Professor of Literature and the Director of the Institute for the Arts and Humanities at Pennsylvania State University. He is the author of ten books to date, most recently, *The Secret Life of Stories: From Don Quixote to Harry Potter, How Understanding Intellectual Disability Transforms the Way We Read* (2016) and *Life as Jamie Knows It: An Exceptional Child Grows Up* (2016), which was written with extensive input from Jamie himself. Its predecessor, *Life as We Know It*, was a New York Times notable book of the year for 1996.

WILLIAM BRADLEY (1976–2017) earned his PhD from the University of Missouri–Columbia, where he focused on creative nonfiction with a secondary focus on literature and medicine. He published his work in numerous magazines and journals, including *The Missouri Review, The Bellevue Literary Review, Brevity, Fourth Genre, The Normal School, Creative Nonfiction*, and *The Utne Reader,* and is the author of the essay collection, *Fractals.*

ELIZABETH BRADY is a Senior Lecturer in Public Speaking at Pennsylvania State University. Her essays on learning to live with loss can be found at mackbrady.com and opentohope.com. She and her family have honored her son Mack's dreams by establishing the Mack Brady Soccer Fund that helps recruit and train the best keepers for Penn State men's soccer.

MARK BRAZAITIS is the author of five books of short stories, including *Truth Poker*, winner of the Autumn House Prize for Fiction, and *The River of Lost Voices: Stories from Guatemala*, winner of the Iowa Short Fiction Award. He is also the author of a collection of poems, *The Other Language*, which won the ABZ Poetry Prize. His work has appeared in *American Medical News, The Sun, Ploughshares, Shenandoah, Witness, Confrontation, Beloit Fiction Journal, Poetry International, Poetry East, The Washington Post,* the *Detroit Free Press*, and elsewhere. A former Peace Corps Volunteer and recipient of an NEA Fellowship, he is professor of English at West Virginia University and director of the West Virginia Writers' Workshop.

DEBORAH BURGHARDT writes creative nonfiction, inspired by twenty years as director of the Women and Gender Studies Program at Clarion University. She holds a Ph.D. in Higher Education from Pennsylvania State University. Her work has appeared in *Globejotting.com, Sabal: Eckerd College's Writers in Paradise Journal, The Bridge Literary Arts Journal, and Tobeco Literary and Artistic Journal.* She divides her time between Clarion, Pennsylvania, and Fort Myers, Florida.

TERESA BLANKMEYER BURKE is a philosopher and bioethicist at Gallaudet University. Her research focuses on bioethical issues of concern to the signing deaf community, in particular issues of genetics and reproduction. In addition to her scholarly work, she serves as bioethics expert to the World Federation of the Deaf and chairs the National Association of the Deaf Bioethics Task Force. She is currently writing a memoir about her experience of being a widowed mother living in the wilderness of Wyoming.

PATRICK DONNELLY is the author of three books of poetry, *The Charge* (Ausable Press, 2003, since 2009 part of Copper Canyon Press), *Nocturnes of the Brothel of Ruin* (Four Way Books, 2012), a 2013 finalist for the Lambda Literary Award, and *Little-Known Operas*, forthcoming from Four Way Books in 2019. His poetry has appeared in many journals, including *The Kenyon Review Online, American Poetry Review, Ploughshares, The Yale Review,* and *The Virginia Quarterly Review.* With Stephen D. Miller, he translates classical Japanese poetry and drama. Donnelly is director of the Poetry Seminar at The Frost Place. He teaches at Smith College.

BRIAN DOYLE (1956–2017) edited *Portland Magazine* at the University of Portland, in Oregon. He authored six collections of essays, two nonfiction books, two collections of "proems," a short story collection, a novella, and the novels *Mink River, The Plover,* and *Martin Marten.* He also edited several anthologies, including

*Ho'olaule'a*, a collection of writing about the Pacific islands. His essays were published in *The Atlantic Monthly, Harper's, Orion, The American Scholar, The Sun, The Georgia Review, The New York Times*, and *The Times of London* and have been reprinted in *Best American Essays, Best American Science & Nature Writing*, and *Best American Spiritual Writing*.

MEREDITH DAVIES HADAWAY is the author of three collections of poetry, including *At The Narrows* (winner of the 2015 Delmarva Book Prize for Creative Writing). She has received fellowships from the Virginia Center for Creative Arts, an Individual Artist Award from the Maryland State Arts Council, and multiple Pushcart nominations. She holds an MFA in Poetry from Vermont College of Fine Arts and is also a Certified Music Practitioner. She plays Celtic harp in a group called "Harp and Soul" as well as offering music at the bedside in hospice, hospital, and nursing home settings.

MADALINE HARRISON is a neurologist at the University of Virginia, where she sees patients with Parkinson's disease and other movement disorders and teaches medical students and residents.

REBECCA HOUSEL is an internationally best-selling author and editor best known for her books on pop culture published in nine languages and sold in fifty-six countries. Housel's doctoral research included a transnational study on patterns of stress in the oncological diagnoses of women; she is also a twenty-five-year survivor of high-grade malignant brain cancer, one of the longest-living survivors in the United States today.

SONYA HUBER is the author of two books of creative nonfiction, *Opa Nobody* and *Cover Me: A Health Insurance Memoir*, and a textbook, *The Backwards Research Guide for Writers: Using Your Life for Reflection, Connection, and Inspiration*. Her work has appeared in *Creative Nonfiction, Fourth Genre, The Crab Orchard Review,*

*Terrain.org*, and other journals. She teaches at Fairfield University and in Fairfield's Low-Residency MFA Program.

ERIN M. KELLY, an essayist, poet, columnist, and freelance editor, is the author of *How to Wait* (Finishing Line Press). She was born with cerebral palsy and wants to be recognized for her work rather than her disability. Her writings have been published in *The Huffington Post, Upworthy, The Mighty, The Good Men Project, Wordgathering Poetry Journal, xoJane,* and *Oberon.* Among her editing projects is the memoir *To Cope and To Prevail* by Ilse-Rose Warg. In "The View from Here," a monthly column she writes for the *Altoona Mirror* newspaper, she addresses the challenges she faces daily.

DIANE KRAYNAK is a pediatric nurse practitioner in Washington DC. Her essays have appeared in *Zone 3, Lifelines,* and *the Examined Life,* and she has participated on an AWP conference panel on medical narrative. Her essay "Heart Lessons" is anthologized in *Creative Nonfiction* journal's *I Wasn't Strong Like This When I Started Out: True Stories on Becoming a Nurse.* Her essay "Lazarus" garnered a Notable distinction for Best American Essays 2013. Her essay "Science Project" won the 2014–2015 Women's National Book Association Nonfiction Prize. She is working on a collection of nursing essays.

TENLEY LOZANO graduated from the United States Coast Guard Academy in 2008 and spent five years as an officer in the U.S. Coast Guard. During her tenure she worked in the engineering department on a ship and as a surface supplied diver. Tenley's writing has appeared in *O-Dark Thirty, The War Horse,* and the anthology *Incoming: Veteran Writers on Returning Home,* and is forthcoming on the NPR series *Incoming Radio.* She was awarded *Crab Orchard Review*'s 2017 John Guyon Literary Nonfiction prize. Tenley graduated from Sierra Nevada College in 2016 with an MFA in Creative Writing.

KATHERINE MACFARLANE is a law professor at the University of Idaho, where she teaches constitutional law and civil rights litigation. She studied Spanish and women's studies at Northwestern University, and obtained her JD from Loyola Law School, Los Angeles. Her nonfiction has appeared in *The Intima, Temenos, Foliate Oak, Hairpin, Huffington Post, xoJane, Ms. Blog, BUST* and *Northwestern Magazine*. She grew up in Kalamazoo, Michigan, and Rome, Italy, which was personally rough, but has since become a source of great writing material.

DINTY W. MOORE has published numerous writing craft books and edited various anthologies currently used in creative writing classrooms, including *Crafting the Personal Essay: A Guide for Writing and Publishing Creative Nonfiction* and *The Rose Metal Press Guide to Writing Flash Nonfiction*. His memoir *Between Panic & Desire* was winner of the Grub Street Nonfiction Book Prize in 2009, and other books include *The Mindful Writer, The Accidental Buddhist,* and *Dear Mister Essay Writer Guy*. Moore has published essays and stories in *The Southern Review, The Georgia Review, Harper's, The New York Times Sunday Magazine, The Philadelphia Inquirer Magazine, Gettysburg Review, Utne Reader,* and *Crazyhorse,* among numerous other venues. He edits *Brevity: The Journal of Concise Literary Nonfiction* and directs the MA and PhD in creative writing at Ohio University.

KAT MOORE is a writer from Memphis, TN. She was the winner of *Profane Journal*'s 2016 Nonfiction Prize. She has essays in *Blunderbuss, New South, Salt Hill, Sidereal, Whiskey Island, Yemassee, Pithead Chapel,* and others. Her poetry is in *Permafrost, Souvenir, decomP,* and others. She also has short fiction in *Cheap Pop Lit*. Her work was also featured in Mothers Myths Monsters at Theaterlab in New York City.

ERIN MURPHY is the author of seven collections of poetry and is co-editor of two anthologies from SUNY Press: *Creating Nonfiction: Twenty Essays and Interviews with the Writers* and *Making Poems: Forty Poems with Commentary by the Poets*. Her work has been featured on Garrison Keillor's *The Writer's Almanac*, and her poems and essays have appeared in numerous journals and anthologies, including *the Yale Journal for Humanities in Medicine*, *The Georgia Review*, *Field*, *Brevity*, *Women's Studies Quarterly*, and elsewhere. She is Professor of English and creative writing at Pennsylvania State University, Altoona College, and has served as the Medical Humanities Discussion Group facilitator for UPMC Hospital in Altoona.

RENÉE K. NICHOLSON is a past Emerging Writer-in-Residence at Penn State–Altoona, author *Roundabout Directions to Lincoln Center*, and assistant professor in the Programs for Multi- and Interdisciplinary Studies at West Virginia University. She worked in the WVU Cancer Institute in a Benedum Foundation and West Virginia Clinical and Translational Institute grant-funded pilot study of expressive writing with patients receiving chemotherapy. Nicholson also served as Assistant Director of the West Virginia Writers' Workshop at WVU. Her writing has appeared in *Poets & Writers, Midwestern Gothic, Moon City Review, The Los Angeles Review, The Superstition Review, Leadership and the Humanities, The Gettysburg Review* and elsewhere, and she has received a WVU ADVANCE grant as well as a grant from the West Virginia Commission on the Arts. Nicholson co-founded and edits prose for the journal *Souvenir*. She has completed the basic and advanced workshops in Narrative Medicine at Columbia University's School of Medicine and collaborates regularly with healthcare professionals in the Morgantown, West Virginia, area on medical humanities projects.

ADRIANA PÁRAMO is a cultural anthropologist, writer, and women's rights advocate. She is the author of *Looking for Esperanza* and *My Mother's Funeral*. She is an adjunct professor in the low-residency MFA program at Fairfield University and an active member of the travel writing workshop of VONA—Voices of Our Nations Arts Foundation—a community of writers of color. She lives in Qatar where she works as a Latin dances and yoga instructor.

RILEY PASSMORE received his MFA in fiction from the University of South Florida, where he teaches creative, technical, and professional writing as a visiting instructor. He's lived with type one diabetes since the age of sixteen, but he doesn't let its ups and downs define him. He recently launched his own knife-making and woodworking company, *RedBeard Knife & Wood*, and is currently at work on a far-future science fiction novel tentatively titled *The Cardinal's Gospel*.

HUGH SILK, MD, MPH, is a family physician and professor in the Department of Family Medicine and Community Health at the University of Massachusetts Medical School. He graduated from McMaster Medical School in Hamilton, Ontario, Canada, and did his residency at University of Massachusetts Family Medicine Residency in Worcester. Hugh moderates a weekly list-serve of stories written by family doctors and learners called "the Thursday Morning Memo." He teaches humanities in medicine workshops for family medicine residents; he has used film in his teaching of medical students; and is a member of the medical school's humanities in medicine committee.

FLOYD SKLOOT is a poet, novelist, and creative nonfiction writer. His work has won three Pushcart Prizes and the PEN USA Literary Award, been a finalist for the Barnes and Noble Discover Award and PEN Award for the Art of the Essay, and been included in *The Best American Essays, Best American Science Writing, Best Spiritual*

*Writing,* and *Best Food Writing.* In 2010 Poets & Writers Inc. named him "One of 50 of the Most Inspiring Authors in the World." His books include the memoirs *In the Shadow of Memory* and *The Wink of the Zenith: The Shaping of a Writer's Life* (University of Nebraska Press), the poetry collections *Approaching Winter* and *The Snow's Music* (LSU Press), and the novel *The Phantom of Thomas Hardy* (University of Wisconsin Press). He lives in Portland, Oregon, with his wife, Beverly Hallberg. Skloot's daughter, Rebecca Skloot, is the bestselling author of *The Immortal Life of Henrietta Lacks* (Crown). They co-edited *The Best American Science Writing 2011* (Ecco/HarperCollins).

MATTHEW S. SMITH is assistant professor in West Virginia University School of Medicine's Department of Neurology and Director of Neurocritical Care. His board certifications include American Board of Internal Medicine, Internal Medicine, American Board of Psychiatry and Neurology, and Neurology.

BELINDA WALLER-PETERSON is an assistant professor of English at Moravian College, where she teaches courses in African American literature and culture, black feminist and womanist theory, and the health humanities. She specializes in women's health issues, maternity, and illness narratives. She is also a licensed registered nurse in the state of Pennsylvania. Her nursing experience and English literature background allow her to explore multiple intersecting areas of study, including the medical humanities; women, gender, and sexuality; and Africana studies. Her articles have been published in *In Media Res: Race, Identity, and Pop Culture in the Twenty-First Century* and *Africalogical Perspectives: Historical and Contemporary Analysis of Race and Africana Studies.*

CPSIA information can be obtained
at www.ICGtesting.com
Printed in the USA
LVHW092042180119
604426LV00002B/255/P